THE NOW STEP®

MANAGE YOUR MENTAL HEALTH WITHOUT GOING OVER THE PAST

LYN PENMAN

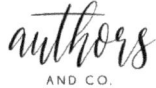

Copyright © 2022 by Lyn Penman

ISBN13 Paperback: 979-8-844043-03-1

ISBN13 Hardback: 978-1-913728-82-3

All rights reserved.

No part of this book may be reproduced in any form or by any electronic or mechanical means, including information storage and retrieval systems, without written permission from the author, except for the use of brief quotations in a book review.

CONTENTS

Preface 7
Foreword 9
Introduction 13

1. Manage Mental Health in a New Way 25
2. The Now Step® 39
3. Your Brain 51
4. Your Mental Wellness Score 63
5. Managing Your Mind 67
6. What's Been Good? 81
7. Sleep 86
8. The Conscious Versus the Subconscious Mind 95
9. The Three Ps 107
10. What Pulls You Off the Now Step® 115
11. The Central Nervous System 127
12. The Now Step® Eyes Open Meditation 143
13. Hormones and Mental Health 152
14. How to Be Solution-Focused 160
    Conclusion 170

With gratitude 177
Work with me 179

For Jimmy, Katie, Robby and Toby

PREFACE

Based on the latest neuroscience, this book will *not* tell you to journal, expose yourself to your fears, or obsess about your triggers. It certainly wont suggest you join a support group.

"The Now Step® saved my life"

— CAROLINE LECKIE, NHS CONSULTANT

"Life-changing techniques"

— JILL CULLEN, CEO

FOREWORD
BY SANDY C. NEWBIGGING

Once upon a time, I found myself completely stressed and suffering... while sitting on a beach in the Caribbean! I had travelled thousands of miles and paid thousands of pounds. I was surrounded by brilliant white sand and my view to the horizon was nothing but shimmering turquoise. And yet, despite the stunning setting, I found myself drowning in dread, despair and fear.

You see, my moment was picture perfect, but there was still no peace. Why? My body was sitting on a beach, but my mind was somewhere else. My negative feelings had nothing to do with what was happening (externally) in my life at that moment, and everything to do with what was going on in my mind. I was 'feeling my thinking' and because my thinking was fear-based, that's how I was feeling.

Although it was an incredibly uncomfortable lesson to learn, I've since discovered that by making the shift from my mind to the moment, I can access more peace, clarity and wellbeing –

anywhere. With this book, Lyn shares her steps for making this all-important, life-changing shift.

Over-thinking distracts us from the present moment. Furthermore, living in the past or future, by over-thinking about your past or future, is an unhealthy habit; it causes stress, sadness, anxiety and even ill-health.

We aren't meant to be 'lost in our minds' thinking all of the time, which is why over-thinking has so many negative side-effects. We are meant to 'pick up' the mind and use it like a tool, only when required, and then put it back down – to work and live in peace and the present moment. With this healthier relationship *with* our mind, and more frequent access to 'the now', we are also able to be more productive, with far less stress.

But here's the thing: we can't get back to 'the now' if we remain unaware of being somewhere else. To heal this unhealthy over-thinking habit, we must first recognise when we are hanging out in the past or future, and Lyn's Now Step Method® can help you to do exactly this.

Step Three of her method involves recognising where you are currently focusing – past or future. By using her method, you can become more self-aware, and empowered to make the choice to return to 'the now'.

I'm an advocate of different tools for different times. I've seen many well-intentioned folks use the present moment to 'spiritually bypass' (and avoid) things in their past or future which require some time, attention, love and healing. I believe there are times when it can be very helpful to step into the past (for a short while) to heal certain things. It can also be useful to step into the future (again, for a short time) when making plans, for example.

However, most people don't just pop into their past or future for a short while and for beneficial reasons, but instead they spend *most* of their life missing the moment. And this certainly *is* an unhealthy way to work and live, which makes us more prone to a whole host of unnecessary problems.

I'm super excited for you to learn ways to let go of the past and future, so you can start spending the *majority* of your days in the present moment. Stepping into the now is most definitely a master key to fulfilment and freedom, serenity and success.

Sandy C. Newbigging, bestselling author of *Mind Calm and Mind Detox*

INTRODUCTION

I see you struggling on.

I see you drowning in overwhelm.

I see you feeling unhappy.

I see you trying not to be suffocated by the straitjacket of anxiety.

I see you trying to stop those obsessive, negative thoughts.

I see you trying to stop listening to that crazy voice in your head, the voice that asks you…

"What if I apply for promotion and they think I'm not good enough?"

"What if I go back into the office and have a panic attack?"

"Why is my boss treating me like this?"

"Am I the only one that can't cope?"

What if, what would, what should, what could...?

I see you lying awake every night replaying the same stories and scenarios in your head.

I see you in the shower every morning planning how your day is going to go when you have not even left the house...

What you are going to say to your colleague, how you are going to reply to that email, what exercise plan you are going to start, what your new tactic to get a promotion is, how physically unwell you will feel before the meeting.

What if, what would, what should, what could...?

I see you in a full-blown panic attack, waking up with that horrible knot in your stomach, feeling unwell with tingling sensations in your head and body, feeling sick and tired all the time.

I see you googling again about the funny lump you can feel in your leg, researching the signs and symptoms of cancer – and yes, ticking each item on the list because you now have every symptom. I see you starting to dial your GP's number to make yet another appointment.

I see you avoiding lunchtimes with your work colleagues, living in fear that you will say the wrong thing to someone.

I see you with zero confidence, no longer able to do your job, run your business or visit your family.

I see you putting your relationships, career, health and happiness on hold.

I see you wishing your mind felt calm, wishing you felt in control, and wishing you could get through one day at work without feeling stressed and anxious.

I see you labelling yourself with 'poor mental health', whether it is anxiety, OCD, low mood, depression, health anxiety, bulimia, or binge eating.

I see *you* – just wanting to feel yourself again.

Going to yoga, having wellness Wednesday at work, attending mindfulness classes, and learning breathing techniques are no longer enough. (I see that you have already tried every one of these.)

I see you and I hear you. I once was you!

I am Lyn Penman. I am an anxiety survivor. I am also the UK's leading solution-focused mental health expert.

The Now Step Method is a new way to manage your mental health and your busy mind. It will help rewire your brain, based on all the current neuroscience and research. It is a new mental health management method that is easy to understand, easy to learn, and easy to implement in your daily personal and professional life. It is a method that manages your mental health without going over the past.

The Now Step Method incorporates fifteen years of personal and professional experience, bringing together all the things that changed my life. It brings together solution-focused psychotherapy, hypnotherapy, meditation, mindfulness, psychoeducation, neuroscience, physiology, and positive psychology. It doesn't bring up the past; rather it empowers and educates you to find a calm and confident solution to the future. It offers you a way to live in the present moment that is practical, not spiritual or 'woowoo'. I promise there will be no fluffy clouds or in-depth words about consciousness or spirituality. Just easy to follow, practical advice in easy to understand language.

The Now Step® is the core of The Now Step Method.

The Now Step® is a technique for keeping your mind in the present moment. It stops you going in the future-where you get anxiety, fear and worry-and into the past-where you get sadness, depression, regret and guilt.

The Now Step Method is a series of techniques and frameworks which encourage you to stay on The Now Step®. It involves you (N) noticing how you are feeling, (O) observing what you are thinking, and (W) where you are currently focusing-past or future. Allowing you to understand how your body, mind and life affect your mental wellbeing.

Some of my clients come to me feeling suicidal, having spent years working with psychiatrists, and are in the depths of despair. My clients, just like you, ready to make that change and find peace with their mental health.

The whole world right now is living this mental health crisis. Do not be fooled by any therapist or anyone who tells you they have the magic pill or the magic cure for you. It doesn't work like that.

I work with corporate organisations who want a new way to manage mental health. A new unique way that gets results and helps them to develop their wellbeing strategy in a solution-focused way.

I also work with individuals delivering my 1-2-1 and group programmes. I can show you how to be mentally well and turn your life around.

I am offering you my hand right now, my hand of friendship and my hand of support. Take my hand and enter my world as I take you on this journey through this book. This is the same journey that I took myself on to help me find freedom from my mind and the same transformation that I offer clients like you every day. If we can do it, you can too.

This is your time to change your life. Through this book you will embark on a new way, a uniquely effective way to help you have excellent mental wellness and to teach you how to manage your mind.

The past is now useless; let's find a solution to your future.

Let's imagine a day when you go ahead and apply for the job without being stressed.

Let's imagine a day when you have no physical symptoms of anxiety, and you go and meet friends for lunch and spend the whole time laughing.

Let's imagine a day when you feel motivated and happy.

Let's imagine a day when you feel confident.

Let's imagine a day when you love living again.

Let's imagine a day when you have good mental health.

Give yourself time to enjoy reading this book. Read it slowly and revisit chapters. Don't make a quick rush though a page when you have five minutes left of your lunch break. Take the time to understand each chapter and put in effort to take on board and implement all the tools and techniques.

I want you to press your 'reset' button right now. Do it: press that button, right here, right now. This is the beginning of something special. This is the beginning of you finding freedom from your mental health. This is the beginning of you having wonderful relationships, feeling motivated in your career, loving yourself, and enjoying living. This is the beginning of you setting an example to your family, being a role model for your children and showing them how to live a calm, confident and in control life.

The Now Step® mental health management method is a forward-thinking solution-focused approach. Yes, we all have a past. Perhaps you had an unhappy childhood, perhaps abusive relationships, perhaps failures and disappointments along the way, (I have had more than my fair share) but we are pressing the reset button on all of this.

Being solution-focused is a bit like driving a car. We must occasionally glance in the rear-view mirror to see if a car is behind us but then we focus forward on the road.

It does not matter what went on in your life ten years ago or ten minutes ago. I will show you how to live your life solution-focused, looking forward on that road and leaving the past exactly where it should be: in the past.

Why are you reading this book right now? Obsessional Compulsive Disorder? (OCD) Anxiety? Depression? Compulsive binge eating? Using wine to numb out the pain of living?

How does poor mental health show up for you? Do you think you feel as an emotion or is it something that comes from your mind?

Do you 'feel' anxiety? Or do you 'think' anxiety?

Do you 'feel' stress? Or do you 'think' stress?

Do you 'feel' depressed? Or do you 'think' depressed?

Take a moment to answer these questions. How do they show up for you?

The reason you are reading this book is because right now poor mental health is consuming your life. You are thinking *and* feeling it. Your life is a struggle, and it doesn't need to be.

The Now Step Method is going to change this.

The Now Step® Mental Wellbeing Framework

Three factors affect your mental health and wellbeing:

- Personal (your life, relationship, finances…)
- Physiological (how you feel in your body, sensations, illness, pain)
- Psychological (what's happening in your mind, worries, procrastination)

These three factors make up The Now Step® Mental Wellbeing Framework.

Understanding this framework will help you manage your mental health and your mind.

This book will help you understand your mental health, why you suffer the way you do and what you can do about it.

This book will give you all the tools and techniques you need to fill your toolbox. These are all the things you need to find the gold that is living from The Now Step®. You can implement them right now to help you manage the crazy voice in your head (psychological), manage your stress bucket (personal), and manage the physical symptoms of your mental health (physiological).

We are used to the idea of getting help to achieve a goal for our bodies. Let us imagine you wanted to become physically strong and fit. Imagine you decided to prepare for your first marathon. You would hire a PT; you would be given all the tools and techniques to prepare you for that marathon.

You would get a training plan, starting with couch to 5k, increasing it so you could run longer distances. You would have a nutrition plan, perhaps cutting out the fast foods and eating a diet rich in healthy carbohydrates and protein. Perhaps you would start yoga to allow your body to stretch and recover. Then *you* would need to be the one to implement all the tools and the training programme.

It is the same with your mental fitness. You want to find freedom from anxiety? Then you must find a training plan and tools and techniques that will allow this to happen. Think of me as the PT for your mind. In this book I will give you everything you need to prepare you for this marathon – in fact this ultra-marathon – that is life.

Empty Your Stress Bucket

March 2020 will go down in history as a life-changing time for all of us. I will always remember standing in my kitchen that day watching our Prime Minister announce lockdown. Can you remember where you were?

It became a time like no other when we were all forced to stay indoors. The world all worked from home and we couldn't see our friends and family. It was a time when everyone's stress bucket filled and the social interaction we craved to help us empty it was no longer available. Our children were home schooled and family dynamics changed. The world's media had us glued to our TVs and the news, absorbing all the fear and negativity.

But all of that is in the past. It is time to put it all behind you.

This book will give you the support and accountability you need. None of us can do this alone. With my support and the understanding that you're not losing your mind, you don't need to be admitted to hospital, and you're not the only one who feels like this, you will be able to make an incredible transformation.

I have been there, I have felt your feelings, and I have thought your thoughts. I am here to show you a new way.

This book will take you through the exact step by step programme of The Now Step®. You will learn about the neuroscience behind how your brain works, and you will go on a journey to understand how your mind works.

Anxiety is caused by negative thinking. You will discover that all those obtrusive negative thoughts that come from your 'crazy voice' are not you! You will discover that your true self is always calm, peaceful and in control. I will talk you through a wonderful mind exercise called 'numbering your thoughts' which will give you an incredible *wow* moment of realisation that we always have thoughts: good, bad, happy or sad. Thoughts are always there but I will show you how you *choose* to stop turning thoughts into thinking. You will understand that thoughts and thinking are two different things. Thinking means allowing a thought to wander into worrying, being angry or being sad.

You will learn the simplest brain training exercise which helps you stop those negative thoughts in their tracks and which rewires your brain to the intellectual mind, the anxiety-free part. Say cheerio to overthinking, goodbye to worrying, see you later to procrastination and au revoir 'crazy lady/crazy man'.

You will learn how to manage and empty your 'stress bucket'.

How full is your 'stress bucket' right now? It might be so full that it is overflowing to flood your street, or maybe even the whole village or city you live in.

You will learn ways to empty it.

You will discover that The Now Step® is the *only* place to hang out! When you have that penny dropping moment and you realise how much better life is when you hang out on The Now Step®, you will never want to come off it. You can use The Now Step® professionally, you can use it to improve your relationships and you can use it with your children.

You will also learn about the why, what and how of sleep. You will learn about Rapid Eye Movement (REM) sleep and its important role in emptying your stress bucket. Sleep is King with regards to good mental health.

You will learn about the conscious and the subconscious minds and the difference between them. You will learn how to communicate with yourself and others to feed your brain the correct positive language.

There is a chapter on the central nervous system which explains why you can get an anxious shaky response and heart palpitations. This chapter will show you that your physical symptoms are normal physiological responses in your body. You will find out about the different parts of your nervous system and how you can hang out in the 'jammies on and chill' zone more than the 'tiger and run' zone.

You will learn The Now Step® eyes open and eyes closed meditation so you can meditate as you go about your day. This is an easy way to get the benefits of meditation without sitting cross-legged in a dark room.

You will also learn about the things that take you off The Now Step®. We will be talking about guilt, judgement, and procrastination. Not only will this help you with your own feelings, it will also help you to understand and manage the reactions and behaviours of colleagues, bosses, partners and friends.

Throughout the book, with their permission, I have included the journeys and transformations some of my clients have experienced by implementing The Now Step®.

I am so excited to share my years of experience as a mum, a friend, a colleague, a mental health expert and, most importantly, as an anxiety survivor.

I cannot wait to share with you my non-fluffy cloud, non-woowoo way to manage your mental health and to live in the present moment.

I see you there. It's time to take my hand. Let's go forwards together and get started on this easy journey to find freedom from your mind and have good mental health.

Are you ready to join me and thousands of others who have good mental health living from The Now Step®?

Then let's gets started.

1
MANAGE MENTAL HEALTH IN A NEW WAY

It is time to turn conventional mental health management on its head. Let's face it – what we have been doing hasn't worked. Look at the people around you. Look at *you*.

The world is facing a mental health crisis right now and it is affecting everybody. Eating disorders, stress, anxiety, OCD, depression, low mood, lack of motivation, workaholism, shopaholism, alcoholism, worry, jealousy, hair pulling, smoking, drugs, nail biting, hoarding, sex addiction, anger.

Everyone is somewhere on the mental health spectrum. Where do you think you are?

The days of being reactive to mental health and waiting until it gets so bad that it stops you living your life are long gone. It's time to be proactive. It's time to start treating everyone human the same and teach them the life-changing tools and techniques of this new mental health management method, The Now Step®.

It is everyone's given right to be able to live a life they enjoy and that makes them happy. A life in which they wake up and look forward to the day ahead. A life in which they feel mentally well. Everyone deserves the right to know this stuff and to be able to see this wonderful world in all its glory. For too long mental health has been managed by talking about the problem and relating it to the past. It's time to be solution-focused.

What issues with mental health do you see around you in your family, friends, and work colleagues? How do issues show up for you right now?

Do you feel sad, down or generally flat?
Do you have excessive worries or fears?
Do you constantly feel guilty?
Do you have low or zero motivation?
Do you think of the worst-case scenario all the time?
Do you have a reduced ability to concentrate and confused thinking?
Do you have mood changes and irritability?
Do you not want to return to socialising post-Covid?
Do you shut out friends and family?
Are you unable to cope with daily stress or life?
Do you feel tired all the time or are you unable to sleep?
Do you lack sex drive?
Do you overuse alcohol or drugs?
Are you binge eating or emotional eating?
Do you feel angry or annoyed all the time?
Are you unable to manage your anger?

It's time to find a deeper way and understanding that will allow you to feel normal again and that will get to the root cause of all of this. It's time to understand the relationship you have with your mind. You can find your solution without talking about the problem.

This book is not meant to replace a proper medical assessment and diagnosis. If you are at all concerned about your mental and physical health, you must always get proper medical support. This book is here to show you a new way to manage your mental health. You can learn how to manage your mind and see once and for all where all those crazy thoughts, worries and the catastrophising come from. You can see what is at the root cause of how you are feeling right now.

Have you ever played the game "Never Have I Ever?" Google it if you haven't.

It is a fun way to get to know a new partner, pass an hour in the car with the kids or play with your mates with a prosecco. There are a few different ways to play it, either by taking a drink, applying consequences or losing lives. You can change the questions to be appropriate to the age group you are playing with.

"Never have I ever eaten beetroot."
"Never have I ever skied."
"Never have I ever kissed a frog."
"Never have I ever lived in America."
"Never have I ever kissed someone of the same sex."

You get my drift.

In this first chapter we are going to play my version... the Mental Health Expert's version. Are you ready?

Never *will* I ever...take you back over your past.
Never *will* I ever...encourage you to tell me drama.
Never *will* I ever...email you suggesting you take a bath or a walk.
Never *will* I ever...tell you to journal.
Never *will* I ever...suggest you join a support group.
Never *will* I ever...make you face your fears and expose you to them.
Never *will* I ever...look at your triggers.
Never *will* I ever...say it's in your genetics.
Never *will* I ever...blame your parents.
Never *will* I ever...allow you to talk negatively.

The reason is that these things *do not work*.

Look back over the list. How many of these things have you tried already? How many things have not worked? Perhaps they made you feel better for a few days or weeks but then you were back to where you started, ramming food into your mouth, worrying non-stop or feeling so low you didn't want to get out of bed.

There is so much about mental health management that doesn't make sense and that doesn't give you the solution. The Now Step® mental health management method is solution-focused.

Let's examine conventional counselling therapy, as an example....

For eight weeks, twenty weeks, even two years, you go into your past at every appointment, blaming your dad's drinking, or the fact your gran fed you too many sweets. You try to find the answer for your past trauma and the reason you sabotage every new relationship you have. You drudge through all the past pain.

Then there is regression therapy... let's close your eyes and hypnotise you back into your childhood home. What do you see? What is making you cry? Hold the bus right there. Stop. Just *stop*.

Do this for a minute. Think back to a conversation you have had this week with your best pal about a past event. You were moaning. You were talking negatively. You were talking about how much your husband's mum has annoyed you or how rude your boss was to you, telling them *all* about it in fine detail.

Take yourself back there right now. How did you feel? What emotions were in your body? What were your facial expressions? What was your pal saying back? How did they look and act? Tense, agitated and angry, I bet.

How do you feel right now, playing that event back? Not great? Sad? Anxious? When we go back over our past, we relive the event. We go through it all over again.

The mind is the most incredible machine, but it is stupid in that particular way. It can't make a distinction between what is real and what is imagined. So, counselling sessions and sessions that take you back over your past make you feel worse rather than better. That conversation with your best mate did the same. The conversation with your colleague about what happened yesterday, that did the same too. Stop talking about your painful past, whether it is ten years ago or ten minutes ago. You are the one that chooses which conversations you have with people. Make sure you choose them wisely.

We are brought up to believe that to live a mentally well future we must heal our past. We must talk about it. This is just not true. Your mind has its way to work through past trauma and events without you ever going back there. This is by way of Rapid Eye Movement sleep.

And that's why journaling (unless it's positive and gratitude-based) is the worst thing for your mental health. Every night before you go to bed you relive the day's events and write down how bad you felt and how much you hate your life. Many people who work with me tell me their past therapist suggested that they read back old journals to see how far they have come.

Stick pins in my eyes right now. Why would you want to go back over that again? Please no, just *no*. Don't do it. If you want to do anything with old journals, burn them, bin them but do *not* go back over them.

Then there is the standard advice on a lot of websites when you google how to manage anxiety, OCD or binge eating. It will tell you to join a support group. Yes, it is important to get support when you are struggling with your mental health, but that must be from people who are positive and solution-focused.

Chances are there will be a few among the people who rock up to a support class, but there may be more who are there to talk about the problem and to moan about how much it affects their life. Why would you want to spend an hour at an OCD support group talking about your OCD for an hour, discussing your triggers and the upset they cause in your life?

Find yourself a supportive friend to go to the cinema or play tennis with. Join a singing class or a walking group. Spend an hour or two away from the problem. The rest of your week right now is filled with anxiety, depression, OCD or binge eating. Please don't join a support group and spend yet another hour of your precious time talking about the problem.

It's time to be solution-focused. It's time to do things a new way.

Let me share with you how I became the UK's leading solution-focused mental health expert.

I started my career as a midwife before working as a key accounts manager for a large organisation.

My journey with poor mental health began when I was working within the fast-paced sales environment of a large pharmaceutical company. It was back in those days when there was zero support from the company and mental health was not talked about. I was petrified to fly to company training dates. The thought of being asked to present in a meeting or speak on stage gave me a panic attack. I dreaded company conferences and would often make excuses to stay in my hotel room. It was a difficult time emotionally and mentally.

When I fell pregnant with my first child, the company offered, and I took, voluntary redundancy. I went on to have four children within six years. I thought working in the corporate world was hard work – try bringing up four children!

I experienced first-hand the effects of burnout, stress and anxiety.

I tried to overcome this period of my life through various therapies, reading every book under the sun, learning how to meditate, attending courses, and studying to educate myself about how the mind and body work. I tried cognitive-behavioural therapy (CBT), neuro-linguistic Programming (NLP), regression therapy, psychodynamic therapy (you name it, I tried it). And then I can across solution-focused therapy. In it I found something that worked. It was a wonderful way to manage my mental health without drudging through my past. I loved it.

Absolutely blown away with the massive change to my life, I decided to make it make it my mission to share my knowledge, training and life-changing techniques with others, and trained as a solution-focused therapist myself. I would help people to stop going over the past and to find a solution to the future.

What a revelation. Goodbye delivering babies, corporate world no more, cheerio to being a stay-at-home mum (after ten years I had done my stint) and hello to developing my own unique mental health management method called The Now Step®.

When I was struggling with my mental health, I was very good at hiding it. No one understood. No one got me.

I wouldn't let my mum take my children out for a walk, and a trip in the car had me visualising the road she would crash on and the actual tree she would hit. Then the thoughts would start playing in my head again and the vicious circle went on and on. On the outside I was smiling and looking like I was loving being a mum when on the inside I was petrified, I was consumed, and I was so frightened.

I would put my children to bed at night and imagine that they would die in their sleep. The minute I kissed them goodnight my crazy mind would start future projecting and playing out the funeral scene. I imagined the state I would be in, who would be there beside me, what I would wear, what teddy they would like in their coffin, and I would hear my screams as if I was living through my precious babies' funerals. Then I thought that I must be thinking this to prepare myself, because they are going to die.

When my third was born I lived with my then husband in a lovely little cottage on his family farm. The cottage was joined on to his sister's cottage next door, and we shared a garden. I remember being petrified to let my two- and three-year-olds out into the garden in case they happened to climb the five-foot wall, or they got lost behind one of the bushes, or aliens came down and abducted them.

Again, my 'crazy lady' was in full flow, thinking *what if, what should, what could?*

Every single night my husband would arrive back from work and I would plead with him to fence off the patio, just a small area so I could open the back door, let them out and know they would be safe. He didn't get it. He didn't get anxiety. He didn't get me. He kept saying no because it made no sense to him, and it made me more and more anxious.

Eventually he gave in. On Google maps you can see the fenced off safe garden. Sitting inside it is me drinking a glass of wine. (I admit it, I drank wine at lunchtime and when I was breast-feeding.)

On the outside I loved being a mum. On the inside I was alone, I was scared, and anxiety consumed me. Looking back on that photograph brings back to me my harrowing journey with anxiety and just how much it took away from my life. It reminds me of the toll it took on my relationship and the precious days, weeks and years it stole from my early times as a mummy.

And the funny thing is, when I meet people who knew me back then they always say, "But Lyn, you always looked so happy on the outside. You were always smiling."

One day I took my four kids to the park in the car. They were three months, two years, five years, and six years old. I was so gripped with anxiety and so overwhelmed that I couldn't get out the car. I was playing out worst-case scenarios about one of my kids running away or one of them needing the toilet and I was so fearful and upset.

I decided to drive to another smaller park thinking I would feel safer there, but as I got closer and the kids continued to shout and cry, my anxiety went into overdrive. I remember pulling into that car park and sobbing uncontrollably, knowing I couldn't get out there either. I was broken. And I was so frightened. I knew then that what I was experiencing wasn't okay and I needed help and support.

I then went on a journey over three years trying to find the answer to my anxiety.

I was in a very discontented and unsupportive marriage. The relationship played a big part in how bad my mental health was.

Bringing up four children on my own was full on and hard work. At times it took me emotionally and mentally to places I never thought possible. But like any parent, the love you have for your children makes anything possible. They were my world and my everything. And every day I got myself up, dusted myself off and lived for my children. I loved them and all the moments of happiness and joy they brought to me.

I was constantly looking to someone else to give me the solution to managing my anxiety. I always wanted a new therapist or a new book. I think I have read every book ever published about anxiety! I looked for someone to give me the answer. I looked for a way to fix myself and my mental health. I was so fixated on the problem that I couldn't be solution-focused. My mental health and anxiety took over my life. Every day I tried to find the answer.

Little did I know that I already had the answer. I already had the solution. The solution was inside me. I was the solution.

I was in Yorkshire on a meditation weekend retreat when it all came to me. It was the first weekend I had ever been away from my children. I remember driving to the retreat feeling physically and mentally unwell with anxiety. My mind was in turmoil about leaving them and feeling guilty for having a break. I nearly turned and went back home on two occasions, but something was pulling me to go.

It was held in a community centre beside the quaintest village green. It was the second day, and everyone was meditating. The room was quiet. They all had their eyes shut and were in their own blissful place.

I couldn't settle during that session. My eyes kept pinging open. I remember looking out the large windows to the green. There was this large old tree gently blowing in the breeze. It had been there for years and years. Despite all the comings and goings of scout groups, coffee mornings and meditation retreats, that tree had always been there. Always standing. Always grounded. Perfect just as it was.

I had the realisation that I was just like the tree. Perfect just as I was.

I didn't need to change. I didn't need to look outwards to find the solution to my mental health. No book or therapist was the answer. I had the solution. I was the solution. I needed to look inwards and make changes in my life.

It all suddenly became clear to me. It was almost like I had spent the past few years living in a busy, noisy, polluted city. People were always coming and going; ambulance and police sirens were whizzing by. Taxi horns were tooting and car engines revved. My mind had been full of noise and distraction. I had been too busy watching other people and how they went about their daily lives. I had been comparing myself to others walking by. I had been going into every store and bookshop to try and find my solution.

But now I was choosing to move away from the city. I was moving away from all the smoke and the noise to live in a cottage on the edge of a peaceful and quaint village where the sky was clear, and the view of the country stretched for miles. Where people walked or cycled around town and there was very little noise. Where it felt like a supportive community who took the time to stop and say hello. Where I felt calm, relaxed and the best version of myself. I was choosing my circumstance and my life.

Deep down inside I knew it was my unfulfilling and unsupportive marriage that was dragging me down. I was deeply in love with my husband and thought we would be together until the end of time. I adored him but had struggled for years and tiptoed around his mood swings to keep our family together. I gave more to the relationship than I received. I gave more love than I got back. I assumed it would always be like this. And because I loved him so much, I was okay with that.

That day at the retreat, questions began running through my mind. They made me question my future for the first time.

I asked why love felt like this. Whether it was really love if I was settling. Whether it was really love if it made me feel sad.

Whether love would ever want me to feel like this.

What if the solution to my mental health was leaving my marriage? What if I deserved to be loved and treated better?

I was petrified but deep down inside of me I knew the answer. I knew it was time to do something about it. I knew that I had to go home and tell my husband of fourteen years that our marriage was over.

It came over me suddenly and I started to cry. I was sobbing. It was a worse pain than I had felt when my dad died suddenly. But I knew someone somewhere was trying to tell me something. I knew I had to do it for my mental health and for my own self-worth.

I sat there looking out at this tree, vowing to myself to make massive changes in my life. I wouldn't be like that tree in another fifty years still standing and putting up with an unhappy marriage or poor mental health. It sent shivers down my spine and a mixture of fear and excitement that I had never felt before.

Over the years my mum said to me, "Lyn, sometimes people in your life take and take and take from you. But then one day you wake up with the realisation that there is nothing more to take. And at that moment you will decide that you have had enough."

These words had stuck with me and sitting in that room miles away from my mum and my children I suddenly understood what she meant. I had given my all to my marriage and there was now nothing more to give.

I had it in me to make massive changes. I had it in me to walk away from my marriage and bring my four children up alone. Somewhere deep inside me I had the strength. Somehow, I would manage. Somehow, I knew I could do it.

It was one of the times in my life when I was devastated but still felt true peace. I stopped going over and over the past. I felt whole and secure. I was well and truly living from The Now Step®.

2

THE NOW STEP®

The Now Step® is the core of The Now Step Method. It is a technique for keeping your mind in the present moment. It stops you going in the future-where you get anxiety, fear and worry-and into the past-where you get sadness, depression, regret and guilt.

The Now Step® is my way of explaining what present moment living is. It is the place where you find your pot of gold, the place that allows you contentment, joy, and happiness.

The Now Step® allows you to show up for life and live in the here and now. Your mental health is defined by this. How you feel mentally is directly linked to how much of your day you spend either on or off The Now Step®. When you live and breathe The Now Step® you feel mentally well. You do not experience anxiety, OCD, depression or anger. You feel calm and in control.

Like many of you, after I had exhausted every therapy, tried five different anti-depressants, beta blockers, and every herbal medication concoction under the sun, I started to investigate spiritual practices to try to manage my mental health. I loved reading books like *The Power of Now* by Eckhart Tolle, manifestation books by Abraham Hicks and others from Deepak Chopra, the Dalai Lama and Wayne Dyer. But reading them caused me stress and anxiety.

They were so deep and so difficult to read I often got a few chapters in and then gave up. A bit too woowoo and fluffy cloud stuff. They were not practical or simple. They took a lot of concentration and energy to understand.

The one concept that stood out from these books was that of living in the present moment. But as much as I tried, I found it difficult to implement this concept when my mind was continually pulling me over the past and taking me into the future.

Meditation really intrigued me. I loved the idea that I could find peace from my crazy thoughts, train my mind to be more focused and resilient, and I could live more in the moment. And I tried it; good lord, I tried it! But even sitting up straight gave me a sore back. My mind was full of thoughts about having a sore back and feeling uncomfortable.

There were so many ways out there to meditate, so many different pieces of advice, that the more I read the more I filled my stress bucket and the more overwhelmed I became. I thought meditation was not for me. Sit up straight and be in the present moment. Sounds simple, right? Well, not for me. The more I tried, the harder it felt. The more I tried, the busier my mind became. The more I tried to be present, the more my mind thought about the day my dad died, and about my son starting school in the future, and about my mental health getting worse, and about my marriage collapsing and having nowhere to live.

Meditation and present moment living made me feel worse rather than better. I was desperate and still searching for the solution.

Looking back, I realise that I was trying to implement all these gurus' techniques without understanding the science, the physiology, and the psychology behind them all. I was too busy trying to manage my mental health and get rid of my past and future thoughts. I was missing the point. I was trying to learn the *how*. I was missing the understanding and the knowledge of the *why*. It was just like trying to get into a car and drive without having any lessons. I was trying to manage my mind without understanding how my mind works.

To this day I am baffled by the number of intelligent, educated men and women who work with me either through organisations and businesses or who find me online and work with me privately and have spent years in therapy, years trying to find the reason for the way they feel. They have been trying to find a way to live without anxiety, depression, OCD, health anxiety, bulimia. They have been going over the past time and time again, regurgitating past experiences, looking for answers.

The solution to your current mental health does not come from your past. It comes from being able to manage your mind and live from The Now Step®.

What about you? What have you studied and learned in the past twelve months? What business books have you read and which seminars have you signed up for? What support have you already tried to manage your mental health? Have you always tried to improve your professional skills and development yet neglected the one thing that can change your relationship with your mental health and change your relationship with others?

Mind management is the one thing that can allow you to eat one biscuit and not devour the box, the one thing that stops you second guessing yourself, the one thing that doesn't have you googling for health conditions, the one thing that stops your OCD, the one thing that allows you the confidence to get on a plane or apply for the promotion, the one thing that makes relationships with colleagues easy, the one thing that allows you to get a full night's sleep, the one thing that allows you to go for a massage and not spend the whole time chattering away to your crazy voice in your head.

It is the one thing that allow you to have peace with your mind and your thoughts. It is the one thing that gives you contentment and happiness.

It is the one thing that has been missing this whole time you have been trying so hard to manage your mental health and feel normal again.

Mind management means learning how to manage your mind. You can manage that mind that tells you that you are useless, that mind that doesn't want you to get out of bed in the morning, that mind that has you obsessively and compulsively repeating behaviours, that mind that has you waking up with anxiety and dreading your upcoming day at work.

You know the mind I mean? I call that part of you the crazy man or crazy lady mind. It is always there, always in charge and ruining your day.

That mind is no different from the mind that makes you dream at night. But you don't have a dream about running away with your next-door neighbour's wife then actually pack your bags and go through and knock on their door the next day.

Yet you allow your mind to constantly take you into the past and take you into the future. It is in the shower with you in the morning. It is with you when you are driving the car. It is with you when you are out for a walk. It is that constant negative narrative that you have allowed to control your life so far. You have allowed it to stop you living in the present moment.

Do you know how the present moment of calmness and contentment feels? The place where OCD and poor mental health do not exist? The place where you love yourself conditionally, where you are perfect and whole exactly as you are?

I used to be an intellectual well-educated woman who didn't have a clue about managing my mind and about staying in the present moment. My life was plagued with anxiety, fear and worry. And reading the books by those wonderful gurus was making me even more confused and my mind even more busy.

My first weekend learning meditation in Edinburgh was the very first steppingstone on my journey to managing my mental health and loving living again. It all started to fall into place for me. If you like, I got my calling. I found my path and my flow to helping others.

Finding the strength to leave my marriage was just the beginning of a very new and different life for me. I had been a stay-at-home mum for ten years but now I had to look at my career and work out how I was going to support myself and my children.

I always wanted to work with people. It is deep within my core values to be able to serve and support others. It wasn't an option to go back and return to my first job as a midwife due to the shift patterns and having four kids. Nor was it an option to go back into the corporate world.

I wanted to show others how to manage their mental health. I wanted to share my story to help inspire others. I didn't want anyone else suffering and wasting their precious life like I had.

I knew I wanted to find a qualification that I could use alongside all the spiritual lessons and tools I had learned. Something tangible yet simple. Something that didn't go over the past but encouraged people to live in the present moment. Something that didn't focus on the problem. Training as a solution-focused psychotherapist was in line with all my beliefs and values regarding present day living. Solution-focused therapy is life changing.

It was such a revelation to find this new way to manage my crazy mind. It allowed me to help others and become the mental health expert that I am today.

I knew I was about to set a new pathway to manage mental health. It would be a new way that did not go over the past and that would allow me to train my clients to be solution-focused and to manage their minds. It was a revelation. After years of searching I now had the solution.

The Now Step® was born during a session with one of my clients.

Hannah had come to see me with crippling anxiety and suicidal thoughts after losing one of her twins due to twin-to-twin transfusion at 27 weeks' gestation. She was pregnant again and was struggling to manage her business and day-to-day life due to the fear and constant anxiety. She was referred to see me by the midwife sonographer at the local baby scanning clinic.

We were talking about her son and whether the naughty step was a good way to manage a toddler's behaviour. I said to her, "Children don't see it as being on the naughty step; they see it as being on the now step."

They are on a step, very much in the present moment. They are not worrying about the past or the future. It's us who suffer because we feel guilty and sad and anxious because we have put them there. We are not on The Now Step.

The Now Step! After all these years of trying to find an easy way to explain present moment living and all the things these gurus were writing about, I had found my solution. And so The Now Step® was born.

It was a simple yet life-changing explanation and tool for present day living. It was a tool that children had down to a tee, that they did naturally, yet we adults had no concept or no understanding of. I had found the final piece of my jigsaw.

I was able to educate my clients about the psychology, physiology and neuroscience of mental health. I was able to use solution-focused questions to help them, I was able to teach them how to manage their minds and now I had the solution and the core premise to help them easily understand it and put it into practice.

The Now Step® is a place where we can be childlike again. I remember putting my son to bed one night when he was four years old. We had just watched *The Lion King* and were singing *Hakuna Matata* as he climbed into bed. He looked up at me with his big eyes and said, "Mummy, I don't get what the song means. Why would anyone have worries?"

It made me smile so much at the innocence of childhood when worries just don't exist, when we have no mental health issues, when we have no fear, worry or sadness. It is so simple yet so life-changing. It has become the core of all my teachings, the core of people living with better mental health. It is the solution that has helped thousands of my clients in the therapy room, online and in my membership.

The Now Step® is the solution to your mental health and managing your mind.

Hannah worked with me for eight weeks and then joined my membership-The Female Mind Retreat. She is still in there making me smile and being a supportive member to others. She truly is one of life's diamonds.

This is what Hannah has to say about The Now Step®;

> "It really grounded me and kept me living in the moment. A lot of my trauma was in the past and although I never want to forget about my son, I couldn't change what happened, so I needed to find a way to stop reliving it. My

thoughts were always 100mph which also made me think too much ahead of myself. It caused me so much anxiety. It was all a vicious circle. The Now Step® mental health management method changed my life and the way I manage my anxiety."

— HANNAH

Let me explain The Now Step® in more detail.

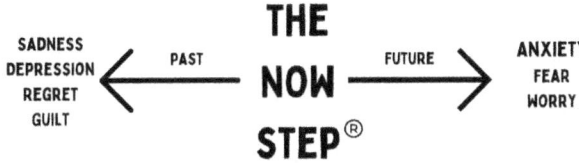

I want you to imagine yourself sitting on a step. The step has N-O-W written on it. Imagine that I come along with a massive, big stamp with N-O-W written on it and stamp it to your backside.

You are now on The Now Step®. Agreed?

Take a moment to imagine yourself firmly on The Now Step®. The problem is that your mind doesn't live on The Now Step®. Therefore, you end up with ongoing mental health issues. The nature of your mind wants to take you into the past or the future.

You might step *forwards* off the Now Step® into the future...

an hour from now, playing out the conversation you are about to have with your boss.

a week from now, future projecting about what is going to go wrong with your project deadline.

a month from now, stressing about the surprise party you have planned for your partner.

a year from now, imagining the worst-case scenario regarding paying bills or your children moving to university.

With your mind in the future, you will only ever feel worry, fear and anxiety.

Similarly, when you step *backwards* off The Now Step® into the past...

an hour ago, annoyed with yourself about the way you spoke to an employee.

a week ago, feeling you let yourself down when you pitched to an important client.

a month ago, replaying the last conversation you had with your dad.

a year ago, replaying memories from a relationship that has broken down or about a family member you have lost.

With your mind in the past, you will only ever feel sadness, regret, guilt, and depression.

It's the way your mind works. It's the emotions and feelings you get when you are off The Now Step®.

By learning how to manage your mind and your thoughts to stay on The Now Step®, where obsessive thinking, fear, anxiety, guilt and sadness no longer exist, you will find freedom from your mental health issues, unwanted habits, and compulsive behaviours.

Where do you spend most of your time? In the past? Or do you spend more time in the future? Do you feel anxiety, fear and worry most of the time? Or do you feel sadness, regret and guilt? Or maybe you switch between them both?

Whenever you are in the past or the future you are not on The Now Step®. When you are off The Now Step® you are filling your stress bucket. When you are off The Now Step® your mental health is not good.

When you are off The Now Step® you think you *are* anxiety, you *are* fear, you *are* OCD, you *are* depression, you *are* your binge eating disorder.

Let this sink in for just a moment.

Your mental health is not a result of your past, it's not a result of your genetics and it's certainly not a result of you being a failure. It's a result of you not understanding how to manage your mind.

It is a result of you spending 99% of your day off The Now Step®.

You are perfect and whole just as you are. But right now, all your attention is going on the past and the future and not the present. Not being on The Now Step®.

In Chapter Three you'll begin to find out the *why* of The Now Step®.

You can find out *why* you need to live from The Now Step® to achieve freedom from your mental health.

You can discover why you need to understand the neuroscience of how your brain works, why you need to understand psychology, subconscious versus conscious, the nervous system, and how to be solution-focused.

Most importantly, you'll learn *why* the only place to live is from The Now Step®.

3
YOUR BRAIN

Let's talk about your brain, that complex machine that oversees all your thoughts, feelings, and emotions. Some refer to it as your mind. Let's start by understanding the basics and how you are going to use your understanding of the brain to live from The Now Step®.

This is a really easy way to get to know how your mind works. It will help you understand your mental health, why you feel the way you do at times and what you can do about it. The exciting thing is that you will be able to use this knowledge to understand why your manager or your partner behaves the way they do. You can understand why they often react with anger or point the finger. You will know why your best pal sometimes hides away, and why your mum is constantly negative and fearful. You will recognise and notice it with friends and colleagues. It will allow you to manage relationships and all the dramas that everyday life throws at you. Most importantly, you will be clear about the role your brain plays in your mental wellness.

This is stuff I talk to my children about. This should be taught in schools. This will help you so much in your journey with your mental health.

Think about your brain as being in two parts – the intellectual part and the primitive, survival part.

Right now, while you are reading this book, you are using your intellectual mind. It is called the left prefrontal cortex, in medical terminology. Throughout this book we will recognise it as the Intellectual Mind.

The Intellectual Mind is the conscious part, the part that allows you to concentrate and read this book. It allows you to be aware of the world and to interact positively. This part of the brain has evolved over billions of years since we became more human, started to talk and communicate, built houses, became educated and became able to learn. It is the clever part of your brain.

We generally don't share this part of our brain with animals. That is why you don't see dogs applying for jobs and cats playing Wordle. It has evolved greatly over the years and is attached to a vast intellectual resource called the Intellectual Mind.

It allows you to look at any situation and come up with an answer based on a proper assessment. It allows you to act. It is the rational part which allows you to be motivated. It is the part that you know as you. It is your true self, exactly as you were born. Just perfect.

When we operate from this part of the brain, we generally get things right in life. It's the positive part of the brain. The Intellectual Mind doesn't make you fearful about returning to the office; it doesn't make you anxious. The Intellectual Mind doesn't make you angry that you have been drawn into an awkward situation in the office again. The Intellectual Mind doesn't let you feel sad and upset. It doesn't make you depressed.

When you operate from the Intellectual Mind you are on fire, you are living your best life. You make decisions easily; you are motivated to have a shower every morning. You are able to speak your truth and stand up for yourself. You apply for that promotion in a heartbeat. You don't eat emotionally or binge eat; you don't allow other people to offend you. You love your life, you are happy, positive, and driven. When you operate from the Intellectual Mind you are on The Now Step®.

Intellectual Mind control is key to good mental health. The problem right now is that most of the population are not in Intellectual Mind control. Most of us think we are, but the prevalence of poor mental health suggests otherwise. Figures of employees with mental health issues have changed from 1:10 to 1:4 post pandemic. As an expert in mental health, I would challenge this number. I believe it is even higher.

Think about your friends and family. How many of them would you say are in Intellectual Mind control right now? How many of them are happy and positive? What about your colleagues and bosses at work? Do you think they are intellectually-minded right now? Are they always objective, calm and rational?

Perhaps you have thought of someone who does not demonstrate Intellectual Mind control and who is making it difficult for you to have Intellectual Mind control. It is hard to be happy and positive when they are constantly being negative and angry to you.

We all feed off each other. We are like mirrors. If you spend most of your time with people who are also in Intellectual Mind control, then you will find it easier to also live from Intellectual Mind control and be happy and positive.

And what about you? The first piece in this jigsaw puzzle is you. Do you think you are in Intellectual Mind control right now? How are you feeling? Are you feeling anxious, worried, angry, depressed? Perhaps you can recognise times today when you have been in Intellectual Mind control and other times you have not?

When you are not in Intellectual Mind control you are operating from a different part of the brain, the other part of your mind – the Primitive Mind.

The Primitive Mind is given to you by Mother Nature to ensure your survival. It is known medically as the limbic brain. It has been with us since our cavemen days and has never changed. Its job is to keep you alive. If it sees danger ahead it steps in.

We all, unfortunately, have this unchanged part of our brains which still operates exactly as it did billions of years ago. Yet life is very different nowadays. We can no longer hide in our caves when there is snow and ice and it's too dangerous to go hunting; we still need to get up and go about our busy lives. When you feel depressed or have low mood and want to hide under your duvet, that is the same feeling that cavemen got all those years ago: low motivation, hiding away from the world, simple tasks feeling like too much and wanting to hide in bed. We have manifested and called this our modern-day depression. In our cave men days this was a normal response.

Similarly, our modern feelings of anxiety come from our survival instincts of being on high alert and watching out for the next sabre-tooth tiger.

Unfortunately, nowadays that shows up as being on high alert and scanning the environment for danger the minute your feet hit the floor in the morning. You worry about the day ahead, always future projecting; *what if, what would, what should.*

Everything is the worst-case scenario and you fear everything. You worry about work, family and yourself. It might show up in health anxiety or general modern-day anxiety.

And it's the same with anger. It is a primitive response to fear. If the caveman was ever attacked or his family or cave was under attack, he would make loud noises, scream, shout, and wave his arms about to make himself scarier in the hope he would frighten off the attacker.

Nowadays we say that someone who is angry has anger management issues. But when someone reacts in an angry way it's because they feel frightened, threatened, and are trying to fight off an attacker.

Think about a time this week you felt angry. Perhaps you felt angry at the way someone treated you. Maybe they treated other people badly. Maybe you felt some road rage this week. Flying off the handle or being irritable can all show up as anger. Is it your fault? No, it's the way your neural connections are firing and wiring right now.

When your Primitive Mind is in charge you have one of three primal parameters: anxiety, anger or depression – or a combination of all three. Perhaps you're not at the extreme of one of these conditions. Generalised anxiety, health anxiety, OCD, clinical depression, and anger management issues don't arrive overnight. Anxiety can show up as worry and negativity, anger as irritability and stress, and depression as low mood, procrastination and lack of motivation. Watch for the primitive brain hijacking your mental health and your emotions and showing up in anger, anxiety or depression.

Do you think your primitive brain is in charge right now? Or perhaps you can recognise that you swing between Intellectual and Primitive Mind control at different times of the day. The changing control is like a seesaw going up and down. Once you start to understand all of this you can choose Intellectual control and begin to rewire your brain and neural connections to the Intellectual Mind where anxiety, anger and depression do not exist, a place where you are motivated, happy, calm and contented.

Right now, most people operate from Primitive Mind control. Perhaps it's not showing up as what we class as mental health issues such as OCD, anxiety, depression, bulimia or health anxiety. But if people continue to operate from Primitive Mind control, chances are the symptoms they have right now (irritability, lack of motivation, emotional eating, overspending, feeling low) will eventually manifest as a mental health issue.

It's time to start looking at mental health management in a new way – that is, Not just looking at it as a problem, and treating people when they show up for support.

It's time to find a solution to make sure we all operate from Intellectual Mind control. In other words, to operate from the Now Step®.

Right now, the world feels like it is constantly running away from the tiger. We are in a constant state of fight, flight or freeze. Let's imagine that you put this book down to go and make a cup of tea and standing in your kitchen is not your partner but the biggest tiger you have ever seen. Cue your fight, flight or freeze response, cue your heart rate going up, your stomach churning, your palms getting sweaty, and you getting out of there like a bullet out of a gun.

Automatically and immediately your body's physiology kicks in, you lose Intellectual Mind control, and your primitive brain takes over. It gets you away from danger. It gets you out of that kitchen. It gets you to safety. It's what is supposed to happen.

Unfortunately, in life the same happens. As your stress bucket fills and your anxiety, worry and overwhelm rise, you lose intellectual control and the Primitive Mind takes over. It doesn't have to be a real tiger in your kitchen but *any* stressful event, be it a pandemic, relationship stress or money worries.

The events in the world right now are causing everyone to lose Intellectual Mind control and to operate from Primitive Mind control. Primitive Mind control gives you three parameters: anxiety, anger, depression, or a combination of all three. This is why the world is facing a mental health crisis and pandemic.

It is not your fault that you feel the way you do. It is the way your brain is wiring and where you are operating from. It certainly does not come from your past. Yes, past experiences and traumas can cause you negative thinking and cause you to go back over your past and relive the event. Yes, past events can make you anxious and depressed. But the solution is not to go back over them to heal them. The solution is here right now, in Intellectual Mind control. It is on the Now Step®.

The cool thing is that with practice you get to choose which part of your brain is in charge.

Let me give you an example of this. Last week I was on my usual daily school drop off with my four kids. There were the usual school morning dramas, with the big ones not wanting to get up and the little ones arguing over which one has more porridge than the other. My daughter was the last one into the car and I left her to shut the back door. All I was thinking about was getting to school on time, so we drove off.

After a very noisy car journey I dropped them off and headed back home. When I arrived back at my house, I noticed the door was open. Cue my primitive brain kicking in with the thought of, "Oh, good lord, someone has broken into my house." My heart started racing.

Before I knew all about the two parts to my brain, I would have been calling the emergency services, grabbing a spade from my shed, tiptoeing into my house and checking behind doors in the hope of catching the thief red-handed and banging him on the head with the spade.

But I know better than this. When I recognised my Primitive Mind kicking in, I was able to stand at the back door and rationalise. I thought, "Ok, Lyn, let's switch your intellectual mind on here. Let's not react. Why is the back door open? What is the rational explanation?"

Katie was the last one out of the door this morning. She had left it open.

I immediately felt my shoulders drop and my breathing calm down. And I went into the house, shut the back door behind me and did not give it another thought. I chose Intellectual Mind control.

Let me give you a second example. I was in Manchester on a training course, two hours' drive from where my favourite Aunty Anna lives. Living in Scotland, I hardly get to see her, and it had been about two years since we had met up. I was in Manchester for two days and had driven the five hours from home. On the evening of the first day, my primitive crazy lady mind kept prompting me to do the two-hour drive to go and visit my Aunty.

My primitive brain was saying, "What does it say about your relationship if you are that close to her and don't go and visit? What happens if she dies in the next few months, and you miss this opportunity to see her?"

Of course, my primitive brain would make me think the worst-case scenario. Over and over, it played these thoughts.

Intellectually, I knew that with the traffic the two-hour drive could turn into three hours. Intellectually, I knew that she was young and healthy, and that chances were she would live a lot more years so that I could visit her later. Intellectually, I knew that I had another full day at a training course the next day and then the five-hour drive home.

It was simple. I had to listen to my Intellectual Mind and stop paying attention to my primitive negative mind. I wouldn't go and visit my Aunty but rather have a nice walk around the hotel, have dinner with my friends who were there, and get an early night ready for day two. I chose Intellectual Mind control.

Do you have a lot of negative and obsessional thoughts? Perhaps these are about weight loss or about conversations you have had that day. They could be about your health or other worries? Maybe you have OCD and compulsive thoughts about things being a certain way, and these same thoughts play on repeat. Have you noticed that these thoughts you have are always negative? Always worst-case scenario?

Welcome to Primitive Mind control. When the Primitive Mind is in charge you always have negative and obsessional thoughts. Why do you think this is? The Primitive Mind is a negative and obsessional mind. Remember that. There is no point in you having a part of your brain for your survival if it's not negative and obsessional.

The Primitive Mind doesn't want you seeing a tiger and thinking, "How cool, I'm going to walk over to it and try to get a selfie." It wants you to think, "Quick, run, it's going to snaffle me." It has to think negatively and worst-case scenario.

Similarly, if I told you right now that there was a tiger in your back garden your Primitive Mind would keep reminding you, obsessing over it, telling you again and again so you don't forget and walk outside and get eaten.

What things do you check again and again? Do you do the social media surf every time you pick up your phone and check it all… Facebook, WhatsApp, Messenger, Instagram and LinkedIn? This is how the primitive survival response shows up in modern times.

Perhaps you check your front door time and time again; perhaps its checking to make sure you have put all the lights off. This survival response can manifest in OCD when obsessive thoughts make you carry out obsessive compulsions because they make you feel safe. They reduce anxiety and worry for a while but soon the cycle continues.

The Primitive Mind is also vigilant. It is always on high alert, scanning the environment for the next danger. It tells you there is another tiger around the corner so you must stay alert. It can make you hyper-vigilant to the next problem occurring in your life. The minute your eyes wake up in the morning – ping! You are scanning the environment for the next problem and the next danger. It can be exhausting. It can keep you awake at night with your mind racing almost like a tiger is waiting in your kitchen. You wouldn't sleep if there was a tiger close by.

The Primitive Mind is also not intellectual. It can't come up with new ideas so it makes you repeat previous and inappropriate behaviours. It doesn't care how much time you have spent that day worrying about problems or staying vigilant for the next tiger. All it cares about is that you have survived another day and night.

We all have a part of our Primitive Mind called the hippocampus. It is here that you save your templated behaviour. Imagine an old-fashioned filing cabinet with files in it. Your hippocampus is like a filing cabinet. If in the past you reached for food for comfort when you were stressed, then emotional or binge eating may be stored inside your hippocampus. Perhaps you get angry easily, and shout and scream, or perhaps OCD or excessive drinking or overspending is your survival template.

Do you have any fears and phobias? Perhaps heights or flying. These too are stored in your hippocampus. Whatever you have stored as your templated survival behaviour will show up when you are in Primitive Mind control. It's not your fault. It's the way your brain is wiring right now.

There is also a part called the amygdala which gives off your fight, flight or freeze response. This part is very much needed when you are faced with a dangerous situation. It is handy when you are faced with a tiger, but not so handy when you are trying to manage your workload or arrange a surprise party for your best friend.

Your mental health is a direct result of the part of your brain that is in charge. It is a direct result of where your neural connections are inside your brain. It is not your fault. Never. It is how your brain is wiring.

The Now Step® mental health management method will rewire your brain so you have more intellectual mind control.

You can take control of this, right here, right now.

Start to recognise which part of your brain you are operating from. Choose Intellectual Mind control.

4

YOUR MENTAL WELLNESS SCORE

You now have an idea of where your brain is wiring to. Are you positively in Intellectual Mind control or is the negative obsessional primitive brain in charge?

You can get good at judging this yourself. Check in with yourself during the day and as events occur. You will soon get to notice where you spend most of the time. You will also be able to recognise it in others. Are they in intellectual or primitive brain control?

But let's find out for definite where you sit with regards to Intellectual Mind control and Primitive Mind control. Let's take away the guessing. These are questions I use in sessions with clients. You can answer them every week to assess where you are and to see where the positive steps forward are coming from. They allow you to be in Intellectual Mind control and find out exactly where you are without any emotion or negative voice from your crazy lady/crazy man.

Grab a pen and paper to find your mental wellness score:

Answer these seven questions using the scaling scores from 1-10, where one is the least and ten is the most.

How much time in the past week has your mind been on The Now Step®? (How much have you been present? How much has your mind been in the past, feeling sad, or in the future, projecting and worrying.)

How positive have your thoughts been? (Have you been chatting all week to your negative crazy voice?)

How much positive action have you taken this week? (This doesn't have to be exercise; it could be tidying your garden shed or finishing off a project, whatever positive action looks like for you.)

How much positive interaction have you had this week? (Have you lifted your head to say hello to your neighbour? Have you had happy chats with your colleagues?)

What is your overall sense of achievement this week? (What have you completed? What has made you feel satisfied?)

How much have you been utilising your strengths? (We all have our own unique strengths. What are yours? If you're not sure, ask a friend. It could be listening, coaching, kindness. If you are not using your unique strengths, then you are not using your potential.)

How happy do you feel right now?

Great! Now you have scored all seven questions, add them up. You will have a number out of seventy.

The average person's emotional wellness is 44.

You certainly are not settling for being average. Average can be seen on the line below in the diagram. If you scored lower than 44 it suggests you have Primitive Mind control. If you have poor mental wellness right now, chances are your score is well below 44. This is okay. This is normal. It is what I would expect. Most of my clients begin our sessions with a score between fifteen and thirty.

MENTAL WELLBEING

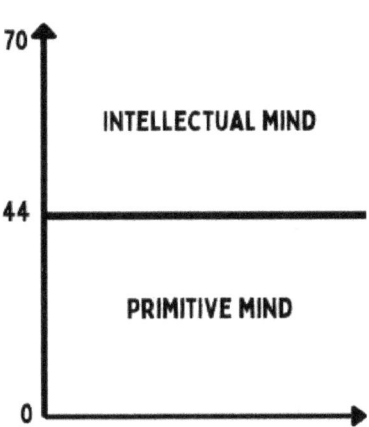

Your score is temporary. By following everything in this book and being solution-focused your score will improve. Don't worry about your score. There is no right or wrong answer. It's simply a tool to allow you to see where you are so you can be solution-focused and find your solution.

If your score is above 44 this suggests you are in Intellectual Mind control. To feel mentally well, your aim is to always score sixty or above.

By implementing The Now Step Method you will naturally begin to move your score up towards sixty.

Just to keep this real for you, I work with clients for a period of eight weeks. It can take six to eight weeks to get your score up to sixty. It does not happen overnight. It will only happen if you commit right now to keeping this book as your little bible, referring to it most days and utilising all the new tools and techniques.

Come back and revisit the questions every week. Watch your score improve.

Making the switch from Primitive Mind control to Intellectual Mind control is very achievable with consistency.

5
MANAGING YOUR MIND

It was 2011 and my mum and I were out on one of our regular day trips to Edinburgh. I had Jimmy and Katie in the double buggy, and they were aged one and two. We were walking up Castle Street which has a wonderful view of Edinburgh Castle. I stopped to give the kids a drink of juice. A tourist was taking a photograph of Edinburgh Castle and we happened to be in his view. At the time I was struggling with bad anxiety and my primitive survival brain was in charge. I didn't see that he was taking a photograph of Edinburgh Castle. I thought he was taking a photograph of my children.

He was part of an internet ring. He was coming back later to steal my children. I immediately jumped into panic mode. I was so upset about it that I called the police. I started to ramble on about what had just happened and how fearful I was for my children's safety. I asked the call handler, "Have you had lots of other phone calls like this today? Are there other people out there taking random photos of children?"

The phone line went quiet. There was silence. Before the woman had a chance to answer me, I had this penny dropping moment. No, Lyn, of course there hadn't been any other phone calls. I had the realisation that it wasn't the actual event of the man taking the photographs that had upset me.

If it had been the event, then all the other people on the street that day with children would have been reporting the same thing. What upset me was the relationship I had with the thoughts in my mind. It was how I was interpreting the event. It was my thoughts and thinking surrounding the event. It was my interpretation of what the crazy lady voice in my head was telling me. Your crazy lady/crazy man voice has so much to answer for.

Anxiety is caused by negative thinking.

Depression is caused by negative thinking.

OCD is caused by negative thinking.

Health anxiety is caused by negative thinking.

It all starts with negative thinking.

It's not the events that happen in your life that cause all these things but the thoughts you have surrounding them.

Think about how the people you know respond to different situations. How do you respond to situations and events in your life? Some people can go through a house move and glide their way through it. A relationship breakup can tip some people over the edge, yet others manage to cope. Some people go through job interviews or a change in career like a duck in water, yet others are crippled by doubt, lack of confidence and worry. It's not the events that cause your mental health issues but the thoughts and the way you manage your mind when these events occur.

When Andrew was referred to work with me by his HR Director at work, he was struggling with OCD and anxiety. Working as a line manager, he was involved in a lot of the pressures and changes that came from the Covid pandemic and working from home. It became apparent that he had lost all confidence in himself as a manager and wasn't sleeping at nights due to anxiety and stress. He doubted every decision he made and felt to blame for the changes in structure that were being implemented by his organisation.

He wanted to be back working in the office. He hated being stuck at home with the noise of his young kids in the background and he missed the face-to-face contact with employees. He found it hard to understand why so many enjoyed working from home. He began to resent them. This caused him to feel negative about every company decision and he dreaded showing up every day to support his team. It wasn't the changes in the working environment that was causing him the stress and anxiety but his thinking and worrying regarding it.

This was just like me that day in Edinburgh. How often do you allow the way your mind interprets events to make you feel mentally unwell, anxious and depressed? Imagine a day when you can ignore these thoughts and show up for life and enjoy all these things. This is possible when you learn how to manage your stress bucket.

Your Stress Bucket

Your stress bucket is in the primitive part of your brain. We all have one. Every negative thought you have is converted and stored inside your stress bucket. Every worry, judgement, self-criticism, opinion of others, stuff you take in from TV and social media, negative self-talk all goes in and fills your stress bucket.

It's not filled by positive, happy thoughts. Those kind of thoughts are okay. It's okay to daydream and come off The Now Step® if you are thinking happy thoughts. But it is not okay when you have negative thoughts. It is negative thinking that fills your stress bucket.

Imagine your stress bucket. Over the course of your day it is filled with stressful events. There's commuting into work, being back in work for the first time, traffic, your full email inbox, that ten am meeting with a very primitive-minded member of your team. Then there is that phone call from a manager saying three staff members are off sick, the lunchtime chat with your work pal when all she talks about is how much she hates her job, the afternoon dentist appointment, the project with a deadline of five pm that is going to make you late home, dinner with your kids, the fall out with your partner, the sink that blocks after tea, the pile of ironing or the grass that needs cutting. All these events go into your stress bucket. However, it's not only the actual events that go in and fill it but all your negative chatter, worries and thinking that surround the events.

Stop for a moment and become aware of what has been going through your mind today. What is going on in your mind right now? What have you been thinking about? Has your positive

Intellectual Mind been in charge or has your Primitive Mind had you thinking negatively about everything? What are you worrying about? What chatter have you had with yourself and with other people?

In your meetings today have you been met with positive solutions and opinions and other people have Intellectual Mind control or have you spent all day dealing with negative opinions and other people's primitive mind and stress buckets?

How about that conversation with your mum earlier? What was she sharing with you? Was she moaning and complaining and filling up your stress bucket? What internal conversations have you been having with yourself recently?

Think about an event you have been invited to over the past few weeks. Perhaps you received the invite and straight away your internal conversation started about, "What will I wear? It's been so long since I have been out."

You headed towards your wardrobe to look at what you have that is suitable. On the way to your bedroom, you noticed the dirty marks on the carpet in your hall and you started muttering in your crazy lady/man voice, "I am fed up with the kids bringing mud in here." "The carpet is so old and I need a new one." Cue the negativity filling your stress bucket.

Then you walked into your bedroom and noticed the bed unmade and your partner's wine glass from last night sitting on the bedside cabinet. And again, the negative chat began, "Why am I so lazy that I didn't even make the bed this morning?" "I am so fed up with John leaving the bedroom a mess and not taking his wine glass to the kitchen." All of this went on before you'd even reached the wardrobe. All this internal negative chatter has filled your stress bucket.

Then you opened the wardrobe and tell yourself, "That won't fit." "Why have I let myself get like this?" "The last time I wore that was at my cousin's wedding." From that point you began turning thoughts into remembering the wedding day and you felt sad and upset because your uncle has died since then.

After that you went back to looking for something to wear. You told yourself, "I have put on so much weight in lockdown I have nothing to wear." "Okay, that is it, I am back on my exercise plan as of tomorrow." "Why have I let my wardrobe get such a mess." "I'm so stressed out with work that I don't have time to keep things tidy." "I hate my life right now." "I wonder what excuse I can use to get out of attending this event."

This started with one simple invite and one simple task of looking for something to wear. In those ten minutes, all you did was talk negatively and fill your stress bucket.

The same happens all day every day. You can think negatively about what will go wrong in the future, and you can think negatively about what has gone wrong in the past.

When your stress bucket is full and overflowing you have no hope whatsoever of accessing your Intellectual Mind. Not a hope in hell. Nada. The fullness of your stress bucket is directly linked to whether you have Intellectual or Primitive Mind control.

Imagine you have a surprise birthday party for your partner coming up. You have spent so much time and effort planning and arranging it. But you have also spent so much mental time planning and arranging it. In the run up to the party you imagine the worst is going to happen: no one is going to turn up; your partner is going to hate it; the cake is going to fall off the table. Intellectually you know that the party will go okay, but you spend every day imagining the worst, playing out the party in your mind. By the time the party happens, you have been at one hundred surprise birthday parties, all of which have been disasters. They have all filled your stress bucket.

It becomes a vicious cycle. Your Primitive Mind is in charge which makes you think negatively. Negative thinking fills your stress bucket and so the cycle continues. It keeps you operating in your survival brain, where your mental health is not good and where you continue to think negatively and see the worst in every situation. It always shows up as anxiety, anger, depression, or a combination of all three.

I wake up every morning with room in my stress bucket. This allows me to deal with the stresses and strains of everyday life with four kids and running a business. In the days before I had Intellectual Mind control, I would wake up with a full stress bucket and be screaming at the kids for spilling milk at the breakfast table, anxious and worried about meetings I had that day, and feeling low and depressed about the day ahead. I would throw the kids into the car for the school run feeling wound up, anxious and stressed. I was ready to fight off that tiger.

How full do you think your stress bucket is right now? When you woke up this morning was your stress bucket overflowing? If you want to have better mental health, you need to be able to keep your stress bucket under control. To have Intellectual Mind control you need to get your stress bucket under control.

Teaching people how to manage their mind and keep their stress bucket under control is the essence of The Now Step® method. You need to be able to manage your thoughts or they will just all continue to fill your stress bucket.

Every day between 70,000 and 100,000 thoughts play on repeat in your mind, going into the future and back over the past. No wonder you feel exhausted. When you do not know how to manage your mind and manage the relationship between your thoughts and your thinking mind you will always suffer with poor or low mental health.

My penny dropping moment came that day in Edinburgh when I called the police. It was my first introduction to just how crazy my crazy lady voice was. Do you have a crazy lady or crazy man mind? Some people refer to it as the shitty committee. Some of my clients have a name for it, like Jiminy Cricket, Crazy Carol or Loopy Lynda. One client called his 'the bam pot'! I even have puppets called the crazy lady and the crazy man that I use during keynote speaking, online training courses or sessions with clients.

When you have a conversation with your crazy lady/man voice, you are filling your stress bucket. When you fill your stress bucket, you are off The Now Step®. When you are off The Now Step®, you have Primitive Mind control. And so, the cycle continues to fill your stress bucket. The key to achieving Intellectual Mind control and keeping your stress bucket empty is understanding and managing your mind.

Counting Your Thoughts

Let's do a very simple exercise to start you off on this journey to managing your mind.

Begin by being in Intellectual Mind control. Imagine yourself firmly sitting on The Now Step®.

You are going to gently close your eyes and watch your mind moving and your thoughts coming and going. Your mind is energy. Just like the way your hair and nails grow by moving so too does your mind.

Set a timer for two minutes and just watch your mind. Just notice what your mind does...

How was that? Was your mind busy? Noisy? Did you notice your thinking mind? Perhaps you were following one thought the whole two minutes.

I want you to do the same again for another two minutes, but this time I want you to watch your mind and start counting all the thoughts you get.

Perhaps you will notice a thought about a meeting this morning or a thought about a noise you can hear in the room. Maybe you will suddenly get a thought about feeling hungry and what you are going to have for lunch. It may even be a thought about something totally weird like when your bin is due out or where your passport is. You may even get a thought wondering if you're thinking what you're supposed to be thinking.

This is not a competition. There is no judgement and no right or wrong answer. Good thoughts, happy thoughts, sad or bad thoughts – they all get counted. Set your timer on your phone for two minutes, close your eyes and begin counting your thoughts…

How many did you get? Write it down.

Now forget all about that number. Focus again on being on The Now Step® and being in Intellectual Mind control. Be relaxed, calm and still. Do it now. Put the book down for a moment and really focus.

What are you going to think next? Do you ever know what you are going to think next? Your mind is probably telling you that you are going to have a thought next or think about what you were thinking before. But do it once more.

The Now Step®; Intellectual Mind control…

What are you going to think next?

You will have noticed that you don't ever truly know what thought is going to pop up.

If you're struggling with this, put the book down for a few hours then come back and start the exercise again. Getting the hang of this is important for your mind management journey.

If you never know what you are going to think next, what does that tell you about your thoughts? It tells you that thoughts are random. Just like your nails grow, your mind moves. It is energy. All day, every day, while you are awake and while you sleep, your mind moves with random thoughts. Whether they are good thoughts, bad thoughts, happy thoughts or sad thoughts, they are always there. You do not control your thoughts. Your thoughts are not you. They are energy moving inside your body.

You do have control over the point you notice the thought. During the exercise, you had control at the point when you gave it a number. You have control at the point when your Primitive Mind, as is its nature, turns those thoughts into thinking and gives the thought a story, makes it into a drama, adds on arms and legs. *What if, what would, what could, what should.* Then it debates, argues, worries, ruminates for two minutes, five minutes, maybe even hours over a thought. A simple random thought. A thought that is not true or correct. It is a narrative that has come up from your subconscious programming, your crazy lady or crazy man here to ruin your day.

The key to managing your mind is not to get rid of your thoughts but to understand and notice them and to be able to live peacefully with them.

This is just like living with the changing weather. You don't wake up, see dark clouds in the sky and assume it is going to rain all day. You look around and see that the sky has some brighter areas. You expect the weather to change as the day goes on. You dress for the weather, taking an umbrella and a jacket just in case. That dark cloud will not follow you around all day unless you let it.

Buddhist monks who live a peaceful, contented life, meditating for hours on end, having this constant relaxed smile, don't ever get rid of their thoughts. Rather they learn how to achieve peace with their busy mind. They watch their own minds move as observers.

Have you ever tried to meditate? If you have never tried meditation, then congratulations – now you have.

That counting your thoughts exercise was meditation. You were watching your mind and becoming aware of your thoughts. You were noticing them but never turning them into thinking. You can use the numbering your thoughts exercise the next time you are in the shower or the next time you notice that your mind is busy and worrying when you are driving.

Notice it, give it a number, let it go and repeat. Because the more you do not turn your thoughts into thinking, the more time you are spending on The Now Step®. The more time you spend on The Now Step®, the emptier your stress bucket will be and the more time you will spend in Intellectual Mind control.

When you become aware that your thoughts are not you, you begin to also have an awareness of your anxiety not being you. How often do you say, "I can't live with *my* anxiety any longer." "I am fed up living with *my* anxiety.'? Just as your thoughts are separate from you, so too are your anxiety and your depression separate from you. They are not you. You are perfect and whole exactly as you are. It is just that right now you are giving all your attention to the thoughts and the worry, the anxiety, and the depression. It's time to start putting all your attention on you.

No baby has ever been born and thought it *was* anxiety. No baby has ever been born and thought it was not good enough or that it didn't like its hair or eye colour. It is all of life's conditioning and experiences that make you think and feel these things as an adult. Think back to that true perfect self of you as a baby. This is the true part of you. It is the one that lives on The Now Step®.

It's important to note that your crazy voice will never disappear. Unfortunately, it is part of your subconscious programming. It will always pop up to try and take you off The Now Step®.

The other day I was walking along St Andrews pier and the thought, "What would happen if you jumped into the deep water, Lyn?" appeared. Out of nowhere it was just suddenly in my mind.

My crazy lady was on my walk with me. I was able to choose. I was able to see the thought for what it was and ignore it. I was able to recognise it for what it was and let it go. I was able to get on with enjoying my walk on the pier.

When clients get to know me, they often share their crazy thoughts with me. As often as not they are thoughts that I have had myself in the past. They are thoughts such as:

"Maybe you should drive off this bridge."

"I can't let my son go on the school trip in case the bus crashes."

"The plane is going to crash, and we are all going to die."

"What if I drop my baby on the floor?"

Take a moment to recognise all the times you get a crazy thought. We all get them. But you now have the incredible secret to stop turning them into thinking. You get to choose. You get to acknowledge them for what they are and let them go.

Do you think you are a positive person? Maybe you are reading and feel some resistance because you believe that you think positively. Consider your thinking over the past few hours. Has your thinking been positive? Has your thinking been productive? Has it been giving you a positive outcome?

You might describe yourself as someone who sees the silver lining to every cloud. Even if the cloud has a silver lining for you, you're still staring at the cloud. Imagine if you could rewire your brain and train your mind to not see the silver lining on the cloud but rather the blue skies behind the clouds?

The Now Step® mental health management method will allow you to do this. It is time to see the blue skies and not the clouds. Silver lining or no silver lining.

When you recognize a crazy thought just acknowledge it for what it is. Then let it go. Do not turn your thoughts into thinking.

6
WHAT'S BEEN GOOD?

The quickest and easiest way to avoid turning your thoughts into thinking is to ask yourself the question, "What's been good today?" when you notice you are away in your thinking mind.

This simple exercise, *What's been good?* is gold dust brain training because the minute you ask it, you switch from the negative primitive brain into Intellectual Mind control. Start making *What's been good?* a daily practice. The more time you spend in Intellectual Mind control, the better your mental health will be.

You don't make a shopping list for a roast dinner and write out the stuff you *don't* want. Can you imagine if your list said:

Don't get apples

Don't get washing powder

Don't get mushrooms

Don't get bacon

Don't get almonds

Don't get orange juice

Your list needs to say what you do want:

Sirloin beef joint

Potatoes

Carrots

Gravy powder

Cooking oil

It is only when we are clear on what we *do* want in life that we start to become solution-focused.

Right now, your mind might be constantly thinking about what you don't want:

I don't want to feel anxious any more.

I'm fed up with my mind racing.

Why do I feel so low and depressed all the time?

I hate my job.

By using the simple question *What has been good today?* you begin to train your brain to see the positives. You start to think in a solution-focused way about the life you do want and the way you want to feel.

What's been good? Do it in the morning when you wake up; do it as you drive to work. If you can't sleep at night, gently ask yourself, "What's been good today?" Before you go into a meeting, before you respond angrily to that email or before you go raging into conflict with your children or partner, switch on your intellectual mind. What's been good? What's been good? What's been good?

Tell your partner and your best friends about this exercise and why you are using it. Share it with them to help them to also be more solution focused. My partner and I do our *What's been good?* every night before we fall asleep. When we are in the hot tub with our children, we involve them and ask them to share. If we have a conversation or a heated debate and start bringing up things from the day before, we remind each other to get back on The Now Step® by asking what's been good today.

It is an easy way to take negativity, finger pointing or blame away from a situation. It is also a gentle reminder that we often get upset by things that have happened and the only way to move forward and feel happy is to let them go. Nothing is worth feeling angry, resentful and annoyed about. The power of living in the present moment allows us to let go of these emotions. My children are brilliant at doing this now and when I bring up something that happened a few days ago, they remind me, "Mum, the past is now useless."

If, like me, you are separated or divorced it can be emotional when your children want to look back at family photos and relive memories. It is painful to bring up the past. I allow my children the space and time to talk about these things, but the minute anyone starts to get upset, sad or negative I will throw in, "Come on, let's think about what has been good," to allow them to have happy and positive thoughts. When you have your family on board you can all support each other to live from The

Now Step®. There are no ongoing arguments as you discuss things and sort them out then and there. No one is made to feel sad and anxious by being constantly reminded about making a mistake last week or last year. Family life is crazy at times, but you can keep some control and calm by asking what has been good.

When you've practised for a few weeks, you can start using it more specifically.

You can ask, "What's been good since I woke up this morning?" "What's been good about work this week?" "What's been good about my nutrition and exercise today?"

If you find this exercise difficult it is because your primitive brain is in charge. Just keep at it. Your mental wellness and your confidence and productivity will thank you for it.

This exercise may sound super simple, but it will transform your relationship with your mind and your mental health.

Veronica works within the NHS and manages a team of thirty staff. When she joined my monthly membership The Female Mind Retreat she had been off work for four months with stress and anxiety. She had seen my posts on social media about a new way to manage your mental health. She wanted her life back and to be able to go back to work and was ready to try anything.

Veronica listened to the modules inside the membership and took part in our daily posts. She prioritised learning and implementing all the teachings within the membership. Her first *What's been good?* of the day is her fluffy rug that lies beside her bed. She bought this rug so she could land her feet on something lovely and soft every day.

If you are struggling to find something that's been good, buy something or do something like Veronica did. What could you add, change or implement in your life right now to make it good?

Veronica is now back working and often tells me that joining the membership has changed her life. That it saved her.

This is what she has to say about it:

> "*What's been good?* puts you straight back on the NOW step. Whenever my crazy lady makes an appearance, I ask myself what's been good. This switches me straight back into the non-anxious part of my brain. Lyn well and truly changed my life."
>
> — VERONICA

When you first begin, it helps to write it down on a piece of paper, in a notebook or on your phone. Begin by doing it a minimum of twice a day.

Once you start to strengthen the positive thoughts in your brain you will be able to use it as you go about your day. Whenever you recognise a negative thought, use *What's been good?* to switch to a positive thought.

7

SLEEP

Sleep is *the* single most important thing if you want to have good mental health.

If you are struggling right now with your mental health, chances are you don't sleep well at night. Perhaps you find it difficult to fall asleep with your mind churning around, perhaps you fall asleep only to be woken up a few hours later, or perhaps you wake early. There is nothing more frustrating than feeling tired yet being unable to sleep, especially as we now have our mobile phones glued to us even in bed. This only acts as a distraction to stop us sleeping well.

Other distractions might include a partner that snores, kids who wake you up during the night, the need to go to the toilet, a sore back, a room that is too hot. There are so many reasons why you may not be getting a good night's sleep.

There are many benefits of a good night's sleep:

- It boosts your mood
- It improves memory
- It helps prevent weight gain
- It makes you more productive
- It can strengthen your heart
- It helps your sport and exercise performance
- It allows you to rest and recuperate
- It's when your body's cells renew

Not getting enough sleep can mean that your body and brain do not work effectively. It can greatly affect your concentration and attention span. It stops you thinking strategically, impacts your risk assessment ability and your reaction time. Lack of sleep makes it more likely that you will make a mistake at work, and you have a greater risk of being in an accident. Health and safety at work policies should include an assessment of how much employees sleep at night and how well they sleep. Organisations should be educating and ensuring employees know and understand the importance of good sleep.

Are you guilty of late night working on your computer? Since the massive change in working environments with more people working from home and hybrid working, there is more opportunity to be caught up in things during the day and get into the habit of working late at night. Have you ever logged on late at night to catch up with work and you see your manager or leadership team logged into teams? The pressure is there straight away for you to also be signed on and working.

The bright lights of a computer or using a mobile phone before bed reduces the body's natural production of melatonin which is required to help you fall asleep. Melatonin is a hormone produced in the pineal gland which puts you into a state of relaxation and quiet wakefulness as bedtime approaches, helping your body with the sleep-wake cycle. It helps facilitate you falling asleep and promotes consistent, quality rest. Avoid computers and phones for at least ninety minutes before bed.

Are you a new mum or dad reading this? If you have a new baby or a child who wakes you up in the night, chances are you struggle with your mental health. Having four kids of my own I have had my fair share of sleepless nights with breastfeeding, bed-wetting and unruly toddlers as they started to climb out of their cot. When I worked as a midwife, I regularly supported women who were struggling with poor mental health.

My own journey with poor mental health began when I had my own babies and now that I know all this stuff, I am convinced that it is lack of sleep that causes mental health problems in new mums and dads. If you are not getting a decent night's sleep, your mental health will suffer.

It is when we sleep that our mind is so clever that it helps to empty our stress buckets. It is during Rapid Eye Movement (REM) sleep that your stress bucket is emptied. The last upsetting or emotional event or conversation that you had during the day is the first one to get removed from your stress bucket during the night. Last one in; first one out.

If you have a watch or tracker that shows your sleep patterns, perhaps you have heard about REM sleep. During the night, you have three sleep patterns: light sleep, deep sleep and REM sleep. They run on a constant cycle. Each cycle lasts about 90-120 minutes. Ideally you need between four and six cycles of sleep every 24 hours. Each cycle represents four different stages, three of which are non-REM and one is REM.

Stage one is the shortest, lasting 5-10 mins. The mind and body both slow down to prepare you for deep sleep and you begin to feel relaxed and sleepy. This is the stage when it is easiest to wake up.

Stage two is the second light sleep phase and lasts about twenty minutes. During this stage your body temperature drops and your heart rate slows.

Stage three is the deep sleep phase, and this is when it is harder to wake up. Muscle tone, breathing and heart rate all reduce further. This stage can last twenty to forty minutes. The duration depends how far through the night it is and how many sleep cycles you have had already.

Finally, stage four is Rapid Eye Movement sleep. This accounts for about 20% of your night-time sleep pattern. The brain becomes more active yet the body more relaxed. If you see your child or partner in REM sleep, their eyelids will be twitching and they will be dreaming. REM is our dreaming state.

It is REM sleep that we need to understand in more detail, because it has a huge effect on our mental wellbeing and health. It is during REM sleep that your stress bucket is emptied. It allows you to wake up in the morning feeling emotionally refreshed and well. It allows you to wake up in the morning with room in your stress bucket, ready to face the highs and lows of the day ahead.

It is during REM that your mind moves any negative emotions from the Primitive Mind up into the Intellectual Mind. This happens in a dream like state, either a clear or a metaphoric dream. Dreaming is a sign that you are emptying your stress bucket.

Think back to a time this week when someone has upset or annoyed you. You have been wound up by conflict at work, your boss, or your best friend. You decide to tell your partner about it.

Someone else will never be able to understand and feel the same way about a situation as you because it's not actually the situation that's the problem, remember, but rather the way your crazy mind is interpreting it. Your partner says, "You are getting yourself all wound up again. It really is no big deal."

But you go away and have a bath and spend the whole time chatting and debating with your crazy lady/man about what they said, how you should have responded and exactly what you're going to say back to them tomorrow.

During the thirty minutes of precious time you're meant to be relaxing in the bath, you have spent the whole time off The Now Step® and filling your stress bucket. Then you head into bed and lie scrolling on your phone for forty-five minutes trying to block it all out. You are still in your primitive, anxious, angry brain which means you compare and contrast.

Then you decide it's time for bed. But you can't sleep. Of course you can't. Your crazy lady/man is in bed beside you going over the thing that has annoyed and upset you. *What if, what would, what should, what could?* They take you back to the event and take you forward into the future.

Eventually, after lots of angry emotions and tossing and turning, you fall asleep. During the night your REM works through the event and moves it from the Primitive Mind up into the Intellectual Mind where you have more control over it and there is less emotion attached. Chances are, you wake up in the morning and it doesn't seem like such a big deal after all. Or perhaps you even forget all about it.

My wee Gran, God rest her soul, used to say to me when I was little, "Things will seem much better in the morning, hen." Now I understand the *why* behind this. Things do feel better in the morning when we have had our required REM sleep.

However, the problems start to occur when you don't get enough REM sleep. When your stress bucket is full and overflowing your REM can't possibly work through it all, so it pings you wide awake during the night. This feels very different from waking up for the toilet and getting back to sleep. When REM pings you wide awake you lie there going over and over things in your mind. Cue the crazy voice and the negative, obsessional primitive brain. It can be difficult to get back to sleep. And how annoying is it? You know you have an early start in the morning and a full day of meetings, yet you can't sleep. You think about all sorts of things from your son leaving home for university to where you have put your passport and why you broke off a relationship when you were eighteen. None of these things is useful and only fills up your stress bucket.

Or perhaps you think you have slept well yet even after eight to ten hours you wake feeling lethargic, tired and unmotivated. This is because Rapid Eye Movement sleep drains you of energy. Does this sound familiar? When your stress bucket is too full your Rapid Eye Movement sleep has a difficult job to empty it. There is too much in your stress bucket so if you sleep too long and have extra sleep cycles of REM sleep, you will wake up feeling groggy.

Getting the optimum amount of sleep may be anything between seven and ten hours. Having too much sleep can have a negative effect on your mental health just as having too little can.

When I work with clients, we focus on improving their sleep and making sure they are having the correct amount so they wake up in the morning with room in their stress bucket. That way, when that driver pulls out in front of you at the lights again, you aren't set off in a rage. Often your sleep will be the first thing you notice improvement in and then your anxiety, anger or depression will follow and improve. Sleep is King!

Isn't it funny that things always seem so much worse during the night? The next day, the same thing will seem much easier. This is because there are no distractions at night. There is only you and that Primitive Mind in charge and your crazy lady/man voice like they are lying on top of you.

What can you do about this? You need to switch from the negative Primitive Mind to the positive, calm Intellectual Mind. You need to do something to distract you and to take back control, allowing you to gently drift back off to sleep.

One tool that can help you improve your quality and length of sleep is a nightly hypnosis download. Hypnosis mimics REM sleep.

Do not worry that we are about to become impractical and fluffy cloud now. Hypnosis is just a very relaxed trance state, like when you are driving and you get to your destination and you wonder if you jumped a red light because you don't remember getting there; or when you are ironing and your mind is away somewhere else. It is not about turning you into a chicken or getting you to look into my eyes.

There are many misconceptions about hypnosis and what it can or can't do. Do not believe anyone who tells you they will cure your anxiety or binge eating with one or two hypnotherapy sessions, because it's just not true. However, hypnosis is a brilliant tool to keep in your mental health toolbox. Use it to empty your stress bucket.

Hypnosis is actually very similar to guided meditation. It allows the two parts of your mind, the intellectual and the primitive, to focus on the same thing. It's a very relaxed state which distracts you from chattering to your crazy lady or man voice. A trained hypnotherapist, like me, uses metaphors and figures of speech which might not make sense to you at the time but allow for positive new suggestions to be made to your subconscious mind as you listen.

It is safe and it works wonders to help your mental health and to empty your stress bucket. I listen to my own nightly hypnosis that I give to all my clients every single night. My kids listen to it at bedtime. It is nothing weird. It is nothing woowoo. It is guided meditation with the added benefit of messages that speak directly to the subconscious part of your brain. If the word hypnosis is still too much for you then just call it guided meditation.

Using night-time hypnosis is like brushing your teeth. You just do it as part of your routine. You put the hypnosis on, and sleep. When you wake up during the night, put the hypnosis back on.

The reason it is so effective is that your mind mimics Rapid Eye Movement sleep when it goes into the state of hypnosis. How cool is that? It helps empty your stress bucket. It helps you to fall asleep. It aids the amount of REM sleep you have during the night.

If you would like to try out self-hypnosis you can download it on my website www.lynpenman.com

Top tips for helping you get a good night's sleep:

- Keep the same bedtime every night.
- Go caffeine free (it's easier than you think).
- No screens for ninety minutes before bed.
- Make sure your room is at the right temperature.
- Make your room as dark as possible.
- Relax before bed by bathing or reading.
- Do your nightly *What's been good?*
- Bedtime hypnosis or guided meditation.

If you wake up during the night use the *What's been good?* question. Stay in bed, nice and comfy, and gently say your *What's been good today?* over and over. This stops the primitive crazy lady/man mind in its tracks, allowing you Intellectual Mind control and to be able to drift back off. Even better, switch on The Now Step® nightly hypnosis download. If not, then find some guided meditation on one of the mind apps or on YouTube. Have it ready and saved so you can find it easily during the night. Just don't be tempted to start scrolling on your phone.

8
THE CONSCIOUS VERSUS THE SUBCONSCIOUS MIND

Our minds are so crazy that perhaps we will never fully understand exactly how they work. There are many theories and so much scientific evidence out there when you start to ask Google. I will explain the human mind in the way that I understand it and believe. This is the understanding that helps me keep my mental health in check.

We can think about what we are thinking. We have the wonderful ability to examine and analyse what we are thinking about. This is called meta cognition. We can reflect on an experience, a memory, a feeling or a sensation, and we can have distance between our thoughts and ourselves. It is like noticing a drone flying overhead and stopping to watch it for a few minutes. We might be curious about where it is going, what it is recording and who is controlling it. We can do the same with our thoughts.

Where does all the crazy lady/man chatter come from? Why do you have this constant negative chatter and nonstop commentary going on in your mind? Where exactly do our thoughts come from? The Buddha gave a great practical answer to this by way of a parable.

Imagine that you are shot in the chest with an arrow. You look around and question who shot you and where this arrow came from. You lie there bleeding to death but rather than find the solution by removing or dealing with the wound or the arrow, you focus on the problem and ask where the arrow came from. You are stuck. The Buddha gives a great example here of how to be solution-focused.

The important thing is not to focus on where your thoughts come from but rather to use the tools and techniques, such as *What's been good?* or the counting your thoughts exercise. However, it is important that you have a concept that you can relate to, one that can help you to manage your mind and that crazy voice and make it easier to stay on The Now Step®.

It is time to learn more about how your mind works and how the conscious (Intellectual Mind) and the subconscious (Primitive Mind) work.

This description of the two parts of your mind is simplified to suit our purpose here. The intellectual left prefrontal cortex area isn't exactly where your conscious mind is, and the limbic primitive brain isn't exactly where the subconscious mind is. The complexity of the brain's structure is best left to medical journals. It also becomes more spiritual too. Do we really know exactly what goes on inside our minds? Do we really know exactly where the two parts of our minds are in our brains?

Let me introduce you to your subconscious mind and to where the narrative from your crazy lady/ crazy man mind comes from. The subconscious mind is your bank of everything that you are not consciously aware of. It is the emotional part that is not fully aware but which influences your feelings and actions. It stores all your beliefs, experiences, skills and memories.

Think of it as a computer running all its programmes in the background as you work. Most of us have no understanding of the complex machine that a computer is yet use our laptop or phone every day. Imagine that when you are born the top of your head is opened up and everything you see, feel and hear until the age of six or seven goes into it. Every experience you have with your parents, perhaps them telling you off or having an argument, things you watched on TV, what you learned at nursery, maybe your teacher telling you off. All these things are stored in your subconscious mind. They make up all your beliefs and values later in life.

At the age of six or seven the subconscious mind closes off and you begin to develop your conscious mind. The conscious mind is rational, positive, makes decisions and is objective. It is the part that is aware of what is happening and what you are thinking. It only has the capability of holding one thought at a time. It gives you all your immediate thoughts and feelings. It is activated when you are on The Now Step®.

The key to being able to ignore the subconscious nonsense that your crazy lady/man tells you is to get your conscious and subconscious minds to work with each other. This allows you to live from The Now Step®.

The subconscious mind is the problematic part. It is always there, always bringing up your old beliefs and programmes. You need to be able to recognise the subconscious mind for what it is and be aware that it is the untrue part of you. It's coming from the past and pulling you away from The Now Step®. Otherwise, you spend all you time engaging and putting your attention on the negative, obsessional and untrue part of you. This feeds your primitive brain and fills your stress bucket.

The anxious and worried thoughts, the times you feel low and depressed, all have a direct correlation to how much attention you give your subconscious and conscious minds. When you disengage from thought and stop turning thoughts into thinking, there is no separation. There is no crazy lady or man, only your true self, consciously aware and living on The Now Step®.

It is such a simple way to live. It is one that allows you to be mentally well and stay in Intellectual Mind control where you don't do anxiety, depression and anger. It's a place of bliss and calm. Of hope and joy.

Your subconscious programming never disappears but you can learn to be in control. You can decide where you put your attention. You choose.

Why is it so difficult then to do this? Why does your subconscious mind seem so powerful? It's to do with the way you internally and externally communicate with yourself.

For example, you decide that you are going on a diet. You fill your time googling the details of the diet you are starting. You obsess over what you cook, whether it is keto or calorie counting.

Your kids ask you for yet another biscuit. As you take the biscuits out the cupboard you say to yourself, "Don't eat a biscuit. Give the kids a biscuit but you won't eat a biscuit."

The subconscious mind does not understand negatives like 'don't' 'shouldn't'. It doesn't understand the *don'ts* and *won'ts*. All it hears is *biscuits*. Before you realise it you have another biscuit in your mouth. Your subconscious programming is at play.

You then say to yourself, "Why did you eat that biscuit? You're meant to be on a diet. At least you only had one biscuit." All your subconscious hears is *biscuit, eat the biscuit* and before you realise it you are back at the cupboard finishing off the packet.

The subconscious mind always mirrors back to the conscious mind

Whatever is going on in your subconscious mind will always show up consciously. While you are asleep your subconscious copies what you have been consciously thinking about and when you wake up in the morning it regurgitates it back to you.

Therefore, it is important to go to bed and fall asleep thinking positive thoughts. That is why using the *What's been good?* question just before you fall asleep and using a bedtime hypnosis are good ideas. They give your subconscious mind lots of positive suggestions which are mirrored back to your conscious mind in the morning.

During session with clients, I use different types of solution-focused questions with them. We use these questions to make sure the client is learning ways to communicate positively with the subconscious mind.

Visualisation is also a very positive and easy way to make sure your conscious mind gives positive direct suggestion to your subconscious mind. Visualising fitting back into your lovely summer dress brings much more success than constantly moaning about being on a diet. Visualising yourself as the new HR director is better than spending three weeks fretting and worrying about how well you did at the interview. Act as if you have already achieved it. You become what you see yourself as.

When your conscious and unconscious minds are out of sync, an internal battle of chaos starts. Think about your conscious, intellectual brain as the CEO of a company. They need to be giving positive, direct instruction to the workforce. Think of the subconscious mind as this workforce. Imagine the CEO takes a week's annual leave without telling his PA or his leadership team. What's going to happen to the workforce? Yes, they will take longer breaks and not put in as much work because they are not being given direct, positive direction from the leader. Chaos would ensue.

You must make sure your CEO (your conscious mind) is always giving direct, positive suggestion to your subconscious Primitive Mind. The way you communicate internally to yourself and externally to other people is so important. From now on, no negativity, no drama, and no moaning. Positive, happy chat only.

The subconscious always does what it thinks you want it to do

Your subconscious is a high performing workforce when it is given strong communication and direction. Whatever it thinks you want it to do, it will do. When you say you are going on a diet and then spend every waking hour obsessing about what you can and can't eat, you are giving confusing messages to your workforce. Your CEO is banging on about food all the time, yet you don't understand why the workforce are overeating.

You might have a similar scenario with setting an early alarm. You might tell yourself you will get up at six am to have a run before work. Cue your crazy lady man/lady voice as you fall asleep saying, "You will be tired if you wake up that early. It's going to be freezing and dark when your alarm goes off." It is not surprising that you hit snooze when the alarm goes off then wake up thirty minutes later annoyed with yourself that you haven't got up on time.

The subconscious moves you from pain to pleasure

Your brain is hardwired to want you to be rewarded with pleasure even in the most dangerous and testing times. It knows that when you feel pleasure you will be rewarded with a release of dopamine. When you have felt pleasure from eating chocolate or having sex during a time of stress or anxiety, the subconscious mind is clever enough to make you repeat these behaviours. It will keep you seeking the dopamine reward. This is fine if you don't mind binging on chocolate but not when you are trying to lose weight. Similarly, its great if you have a loving partner who you can have lots of sex with but not if it's causing you to be unfaithful.

The subconscious likes familiarity

This feeds into the dopamine reward system even more because it makes you repeat behaviours such as overeating or missing your gym class.

To give the subconscious mind other behaviours that it can start to recognise and repeat, you need to create new pathways and stick with them. This includes new exercise regimes, learning how to manage your mind, daily meditation practice and healthy eating.

Research shows that new pathways take anything from 22-66 days to reprogramme. That is why consistency is key with all the new things you are learning in this book. There is no point trying out the tools for two days. You need to be consistent.

Stop for a moment and think about the narrative that you hear constantly from your crazy lady/crazy man. The constant thoughts and beliefs that play on repeat:

I'm not good enough

I am lazy

I am fat

I am so tired

I can't apply for a new job

No one likes me

I will never have money

I will feel better when I have lost weight/got a new partner

I will always have anxiety

Depression has taken over my life

These are all stored in your subconscious mind where they continue the narrative.

What is your narrative? Write it down or save it into your notes on your phone and over the next few days become aware of how many times you hear this repeated narrative.

Let's get something clear. This narrative from your crazy lady/crazy man is not *you*. It is a lie. But you believe it and hold on to this narrative like it's the truest word ever been spoken. And not only do you hold on to it, you spend all day finding reasons for it to be true, debating how you are going to fix it and allowing yourself to worry and feel anxious about it. What would happen if you could let go of that narrative, if you never heard it again? How peaceful and joyful would your life be?

Imagine you and I swapped heads so you were hearing all my crazy lady narrative. You would hear about my son who leaves his bedroom in a mess, conversations about my ex-husband, my frustration at my client cancelling last minute, how badly I want my garden finished for summer and that I want to lose two stone by next week.

You would probably think, "Lyn has a lot going on in her life." You wouldn't start googling *how to make my son tidy his room* or find my ex-husband on Facebook to give him a piece of your mind.

Similarly, if I had all your thoughts, I wouldn't be reacting to them. I would see them for what they are. Thoughts. Sometimes good thoughts, sometimes bad thoughts. Sometimes completely irrational and crazy thoughts.

The way you consciously act and behave is linked directly to *your* experience in the past. No one will ever be able to feel or understand about your subconscious programming like you do. That's why you and your partner react differently to family dramas. Perhaps something upsets you, yet your partner doesn't seem bothered. The way you consciously react to a situation depends on your past experiences that only you have experienced.

But you *can* choose how you speak back to it.

Imagine someone you love dearly who right now is struggling with their weight or low mood or anxiety. Perhaps it's you son or your best friend. How do you want them to speak to themselves? What advice do you give them? You need to speak consciously to your subconscious mind in exactly this same way. Speak from a place of compassion, kindness, and love.

Become aware of repeated thoughts coming from the subconscious mind. Use a technique to stay on The Now Step®. Do not get caught up in turning those thoughts into thinking.

Become aware of the language you use:

I have a headache

I am in pain

I am anxious

I am tired

I am miserable

You are the one feeding the negative stories and words to your subconscious mind. You are the one filling your stress bucket. You are the one constantly off The Now Step®.

That's why people go on about the importance of using daily mantras. When you give positive, direct suggestions to your subconscious mind it will eventually start to feed them back to you. Doing this takes practice but it is powerful in changing your subconscious programming.

Positive ways to speak to yourself:

I am wonderful

I am in perfect health

I eat well to fuel my body

I love me

I can and I will

Life is wonderful

I am calm

Write these things all over your mirror if it helps. Get little notelets and write them down and stick them all over your desk. Change your phone background to your favourite positive quote.

Stop allowing your mean crazy lady/crazy man voice to be in control. Don't let it hold you back from what you can achieve in life and who you want to be. It is nonsense and is not true.

When the narrative is nonstop and loud do *not* engage with it. Tell your crazy lady/crazy man that you aren't listening and tell them to go away. For the next sixty minutes you do *you*. Be perfect and whole just as you are. Get on The Now Step® and do something that allows you to be present. Dance to music, read a book, cook your favourite meal. Do anything that stops you engaging with the untrue part of you.

9
THE THREE PS

When you have all the tools and techniques from The Now Step® method in your toolbox and you are using them every day you may still feel like your mood changes. You might notice yourself feeling low, unmotivated, or perhaps a little worried or anxious sometimes.

The Now Step® method is your life jacket in the stormy sea of life. Unfortunately, no one, not even I, can wave a magic wand and tell you that have all the tools and now off you go into your perfect little contented world. It just doesn't work like that.

Imagine you are out at sea on a boat on a very stormy day and the storm is so bad that the boat loses its sail and topples you overboard. Despite swimming with all your energy, you may go under. But if you have your life jacket on, yes, your little legs will still be kicking like crazy, but there is a good chance that you will keep your head above water until you are rescued.

The Now Step® method is your life jacket for the storm of life. If you don't carry your toolbox around and use it every time you are out at sea, chances are you will struggle to stay afloat in life. Make use of the toolbox every day and you will sail through the stormy waters.

You will notice your mood is better some days than others. Just like the seasons and the weather change so too do our energy levels, our mood and our motivation. Energy moves through our body and changes all the time. Once you start to manage your mind and your physiological response to things by using The Now Step® method, you will feel more in control and mentally stronger.

You won't be able to change this energy or your moods and emotions. But you can make sure that you are aware of your changing moods and energy levels and make sure you are doing what you need to on these days. When you have a few days or weeks of low mood that comes over like a dark cloud, you can start to avoid people, places and things that make you feel better. You might cancel plans with friends because you can't be bothered getting ready, you don't go to your gym class because you can't face the exertion of it, you eat junk food because it makes you feel better at the time. And then it makes you feel even worse. You become stuck in your own head and engage with your crazy lady or man voice telling you to hide away. The things that you enjoy and make you feel good no longer happen.

Motivation is not found in a specific part of the brain or the body. Nor is it something that you find first and then you follow up by exercising regularly or eating well. And when you have a full stress bucket you will not have any motivation. Nada. Your survival primitive brain is making sure you are conserving all your energy for when that tiger comes back. It is holding you back from completing that cognitively demanding task to ensure you have enough brain power to get through the next scary attack or event.

Motivation works the other way around. It's the little things in life that you do such as cleaning your house, cooking a nice meal or going for a walk that then make you feel good and allow you to feel motivated.

We can only ever be motivated when we have Intellectual Mind control and when we have a goal set for what we are trying to achieve. It's a bit like getting into your car to go and visit a friend who has moved house. You add their new address into your sat navigation. You know where you are going. You have a direction. You wouldn't get in the car and just start driving or there is a good chance you would be driving around in circles.

If you want to feel motivated, you need to be clear on your goal and then start making small steps each day towards your goal. Your goal could be something simple like doing five thousand steps each day, or eating three healthy meals and two snacks, or saving up two thousand pounds for a holiday. It doesn't matter what it is so long as you have a goal in mind. When you are clear about your destination and you take small steps each day towards it, this will get you feeling motivated. But you must start somewhere.

This is where the simplicity of The Now Step® comes in. You need to know your goal and your destination, but any time you notice yourself away into the future negatively forecasting that you will never run 5k or save up for that holiday, you just stop, reset, and get back on The Now Step®. No stress; no hassle.

You can be in control of your own destination and move towards it every day without the actual pressure of getting there.

Many people are under the impression that they will be happy when…

I will be happy when I have lost a stone.

I will be happy when I have the promotion.

I will be happy when I am living in a bigger house.

They arrive at this destination only to realise that they still feel mentally low, unsatisfied and unmotivated. Then they start again with a new, bigger goal. Guess what? They get there and still are not happy. Do not let this be you.

You can feel and be happy when you take tiny steps each day. Otherwise, you become stuck in that constant cycle of low mood, feeling tired and that *can't be arsed* attitude. Low mood is normal; it is going to happen to you at times, but when you are aware that you feel like this, you can look at the mental wellness framework and work out how to improve your mood.

There will always be thoughts that go through your mind such as, "I'm too tired to go to the gym today I won't bother," or the way your body feels sore or tired, or personal factors going on for you such as the fact that you haven't been to the gym for over a week now or the fact that you have been drinking too much and eating unhealthy foods. As often as not, the reason you feel low in mood is because you haven't been doing the things that make you happy and the things that make your heart sing. You don't find motivation, motivation finds *you*.

Willpower is exactly the same. When you feel rubbish, it can be the hardest thing to begin looking after yourself and loving yourself. There is so much stuff about self-care and self-love and I am sure you get it. Yes, we need to eat well and exercise. They are so important for your physical and mental health, but how on earth do you begin self-care when you feel so flat?

I have a solution for you that is very easy to implement. You can break the vicious cycle by using the 3 Ps every day, especially at times when you are stuck in low mood and don't see a way out.

The three Ps remind you of your daily goal and remind you of your why. They are another tool, just like your *What's been good?* and your nightly hypnosis. You can make them part of your routine, like brushing your teeth. Because you have done it for so long, brushing your teeth in the morning or before bed is a subconscious action. You just do it. You don't overthink it or chat to your crazy lady or man. You do these things naturally and subconsciously. By using the three Ps your self-care and self-love will start to become natural and easy too.

The three Ps stand for *positive* action and *positive* interaction which lead to *positive* thinking.

An example of the three Ps is going to the garden centre in late spring and asking for advice on which plants to buy for my summer pots. Then I buy the pots, compost and plants and head home to plant them. There is so much positive action and interaction right there. Then every time I walk past the plant pots or go into the garden to water them, I have lots of happy and positive thoughts about my great effort and about how lovely they look.

When people struggle with their mental health, they are not doing any daily positive action, interaction or thinking. No wonder they feel so low. Think about something you have done in the past that has given you the three Ps: *positive* action, *positive* interaction, and *positive* thinking.

Scientists are adamant that back in our cavemen days it was the three Ps that helped keep them motivated, happy, and helped them cope with pain, because, let's face it, there was no hospitals in those days. When the cavemen went out hunting for food they were taking positive *action* and when they sat around the fire they got lots of positive *interaction*. I'm not suggesting you start going out with a spear to hunt down your tea, although with the price of food these days perhaps it would be a cheaper option! But I do suggest that you incorporate positive action and positive interaction into your daily routine, because scientists are sure that the same neurotransmitter that helped motivate the cavemen back then is the one that motivates us nowadays.

The neurotransmitter is serotonin which perhaps you know as the happy hormone. Serotonin is a chemical messenger and is essential for stabilising your mood, emotions, appetite and digestion. It also helps produce healthy sleeping patterns. You need it for your nerve cells and brain to function. It's an essential neurotransmitter in the brain if you want to feel mentally healthy.

If you are currently taking anti-anxiety or anti-depressant medications, they don't give you more serotonin but rather block the receptor sites within your brain, which means that the serotonin you have keeps circulating around your brain and body.

To naturally boost your levels of serotonin, you can ask yourself these three questions every day:

- What am I doing today to get my positive action?
- What am I doing today to get my positive interaction?
- What am I doing today that makes my heart sing and will give me positive thinking?

These are three very simple questions, but if you implement them you will have a massive improvement in your serotonin levels and your mood and motivation. When you feel mentally unwell you do not want to do any of these three things, but just like brushing your teeth you must do them. Force yourself if need be. Take small steps each day that can move you towards the goal of having excellent three Ps. Only then will you be truly giving yourself self-care. It doesn't matter at the start how tiny or insignificant these things seem.

They are helpful questions to use when you have a day ahead full of meetings with negative, primitively-minded people who will not give you positive interaction and you know you will leave the meeting feeling anything but positive. They are especially important questions when you are going through a very difficult time in your life like the breakup of a relationship or a family bereavement when your day has no positive action. This is again one of the times when you choose how your mental wellness is. Yes, there may be lots of horrible things going on in your personal life, but choose tiny things that will give you the three Ps each day. It may be as simple as making yourself a nice cup of coffee, taking ten minutes to read your book, or lifting your head as you are out for your walk and saying hello to people.

Do whatever looks to you like positive action and interaction.

Once you get into the swing of the three Ps it becomes a normal daily habit. And then you will have lots of positive things to write or say internally to yourself when you do your daily *What's been good today?* The *What's been good today?* and the three Ps begin to intertwine.

10
WHAT PULLS YOU OFF THE NOW STEP®

Everything begins with a thought. Every emotion, every feeling begins with a thought. You are a result of your thoughts; your emotions are a result of your thoughts. It all begins within your mind.

Whatever is going on inside your head (your psychology) will always link to what is going on inside your body (your physiology) and this always links back to what is going on around about you (personal). This makes up The Now Step® mental wellbeing framework.

MENTAL WELLBEING FRAMEWORK

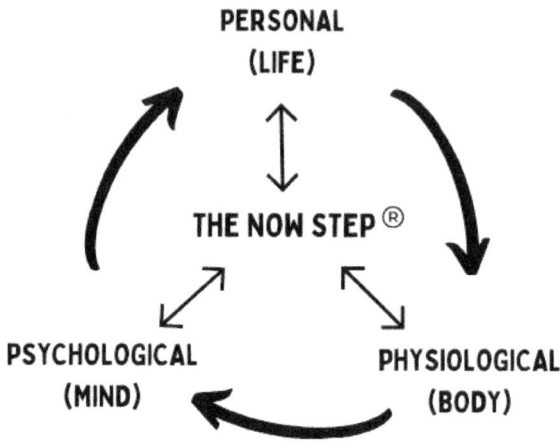

© Lyn Penman 2021

Think about it as a continuous cycle as in the diagram. Each one of these things is responsible for pulling you away from The Now Step®.

Science suggests that everything begins with a thought – with the psychology part of the framework. Every emotion, every feeling begins with a thought. It all begins within your mind.

You have a *thought* which then gives you a *feeling*. That feeling then makes you do an *action* or not do an action which in turn gives you a *result*.

Thought = feeling = action = result.

For example, you have the thought, "I don't have the energy for a walk today." This gives you the feeling of tiredness and lethargy. You don't do your action. This results in you not getting your daily steps in and feeling lazier and more fed up.

However, it might not always be clear that everything starts with a thought. Sometimes you have a *feeling* which makes your mind move and gives you a *thought* about the feeling which then gives you the *action* or *non-action* which in turn gives you the *result*.

Feeling = thought = action = result.

Take low mood, for example. We have all had that day when we have woken up and just felt low. No energy. Nothing. Then it is the feeling of lethargy, tiredness and low motivation that triggers you to start thinking and having thoughts about being low, fed up and depressed. You will wonder why you are feeling like this.

The easiest way to understand it is using The Mental Wellbeing Framework. One thing links directly to another.

When you have problems going on in your personal life or job, it will affect how you think and how you feel. When you feel upset or angry (your physiology) it will affect what thoughts are in your mind (your psychology) and in turn how you show up for life or work (personal).

Do this now. Think back over the past few days to a moment when you felt angry about something. What was going on that day? What personal factors were in play? Who or what was annoying you? Perhaps it was a person or a situation. Or perhaps you were off The Now Step® and you were reliving a past event. What were you thinking about? What thoughts were going through your mind when you felt this emotion?

Now think about a time in the past few days when you felt happy? If you feel really low right now and nothing has made you happy in the past few days, think back to the last time you felt happy or excited. Where were you? What was going on in your life? Perhaps you'd just had a job promotion or had booked a great holiday. Perhaps you were out post-Covid at the cinema for the first time. What were you thinking about? Were your thoughts positive or negative?

Whatever you think about always shows up as an emotion or a feeling in your body. When you have negative thoughts, you will feel a downward spiralling, negative emotion such as anger, sadness, guilt or regret. When you have positive thoughts, you will feel an upward spiralling emotion such as joy, peace, happiness or excitement. Your thoughts create your reality. It is so important to understand this to allow you to live a contented mentally well and fulfilling life.

Over the next few days, tune in to what is affecting your mental wellbeing framework. Using these questions to check in regularly really helps:

- What emotion am I feeling right now?
- What am I thinking about right now?

When you feel angry you will always be thinking about something that is making you annoyed.

Stop. Reset. Get back on The Now Step®.

When you feel sad you will always be thinking about a past event that upsets you.

Stop. Reset. Get back on The Now Step®.

When you are anxious you will always be thinking about a future worst-case scenario and how wrong it is going to go.

Stop. Reset. Get back on The Now Step®.

Never fight your future and never fight your past. Rather, show up for life on The Now Step® and accept it exactly as it is.

When you operate from The Now Step® you are living in the present moment. This is the only moment that actually exists. When you are on The Now Step® you are in Intellectual Mind control. You are not filling your stress bucket. You are putting all your attention on the true self – the part of you that is true and not the primitive ego, crazy lady/man self who is not true.

If you haven't been doing this, it is because you have misunderstood the relationship between these. You have misunderstood the mental wellbeing framework and the effect it has on your mental health. You haven't been managing your mind. This is the beginning of you rewiring your brain and making all the neural connections stay strong in the part of your brain that allows you to be mentally well. This is a new way to strengthen the muscles in your brain.

Just like starting the gym, this doesn't happen overnight. To begin with you will be constantly fighting to stay on The Now Step®. You'll have to keep reminding yourself that there truly is a better way to live. But with practice this will become your normal go to.

Years ago, we didn't believe that we could change our brains. But now scientists know about neuroplasticity. We can make new pathways in our brain. At any time we can begin to change our behaviours and make new patterns and habits.

Think about going sledging when you were little. The first time you made a path down the hill it didn't go very fast. But the more times you went down the same path on the hill and compacted all the snow, the faster and you went. It's the same with your brain. You need to keep going down the new pathway. Repeat the new behaviour.

Put all of this into practice by using The Now Step® and the word NOW.

When your mind is away subconsciously turning thoughts into thinking, and you remember you are filling your stress bucket, then... stop. Reset and use The Now Step® to bring you back to the present moment.

N Notice what you are feeling (happy, sad, angry, anxious)

O Observe the thoughts in your mind (what are you thinking about?)

W Where are you – past/future?

STEP back onto The Now Step®.

When was the last time you were well and truly on The Now Step®? Perhaps it was at the birth of your baby. Perhaps it was last week when you climbed to the top of a hill.

You are on The Now Step® when you have a *wow* moment and the world seems to stand still for a second. Your mind is nowhere else but in the very present moment, in awe and wonder. Listen on YouTube to Freddie Mercury singing Bohemian Rhapsody live for Live Aid in 1985. This is the perfect example of a *wow* moment. Or think about what makes you go *wow!*

When your mind is calm and still, when there is nothing else going on in your mind, but you are saying *wow*, this is how it feels to be on the Now Step®.

Those moments of joy and wonder become your natural go to. The more times in a day you have *wow* moments the less time you spend having *oh no* moments.

It really helps to get an understanding of all the things that take you off The Now Step®. These are the things always pulling you into the past and the future. Having an awareness of them allows you to become an expert at managing your mind and catching out your crazy lady/man when they are trying to trick you. When you notice one of these things you can use N-O-W to check in and bring yourself back to The Now Step®. Become aware of these things as they come up for you this week.

Guilt

If you are a parent, I am sure you experience parent guilt at times. It is that feeling when you drop the kids off at school and feel guilty again that you must work and miss out on sports day. Or the feeling when you remember the angry way you spoke to them last night before bed. Parent guilt exists, but only when you are off The Now Step®. If you ever feel guilty about something, then stop! And use N-O-W to remind you that it's only a thought.

Resistance

How often do you resist things? How often do you say no? Perhaps it's your boss suggesting you take on a new project or your partner suggesting that you invite your mother around for Sunday lunch. How many times in a day do you feel resistance?

When you resist something, you are off The Now Step®. Try for the next few days to be open to everything. Try to show up and accept life exactly as it is. Try to be okay with everything that comes your way.

Judgement

Who or what are you judging now? Is it the way your colleague spoke to you? Or the outfit someone is wearing in a bar? Perhaps it is someone bringing their dog to a restaurant or the opinion of your big sister. Whenever you notice yourself judging something or someone, you are off The Now Step® and filling your stress bucket. Let it go! Let your judgement go and see how much easier it feels.

Comparison

The Primitive Mind loves to compare and contrast. It's how it works.

Who or what are you comparing yourself to? Your best friend? Your team member who got the promotion? Perhaps you're comparing yourself right now with the old you of two years ago?

Social media has got a lot to answer for, feeding the Primitive Mind and continually making you compare yourself and feel not good enough. Stop scrolling through social media. Get back on The Now Step® and concentrate on the here and now.

Fear

What is making you fearful? What are you worrying about? Living fearfully sucks the joy out of living!

Whenever you notice yourself fearing something or an upcoming situation, it's a warning sign that you need to get back on The Now Step®. This is common when you have an upcoming hospital appointment for an ongoing medical condition. Of course, your crazy mind is always going to tell you that you are going to die, or they are going to find something sinister. What's going to serve you better? What's going to allow you to stay calmer? Spending two weeks before the appointment imagining the worst and filling your stress bucket? Or remember that fear is made inside your mind. It's just not true.

Fix it

Is your default to try and fix things? Is your partner heading out for the day and you feel the need to make his travel arrangements and bar bookings? Is someone upset in your family and you have the urge to be the fixer? It is not your issue. Stop trying to people please and fix things.

Past/Future

When exactly are you right now? Every time you become aware that you are not living on The Now Step® and you are either in the future, worrying, or in the past, feeling sad and depressed... stop. You choose.

Asking why?

Any time you notice your crazy lady/man asking *why*, you need to remind yourself to stop, reset and get back on The Now Step®. Any time you question and ask *why,* it is a lie. It is the untrue voice inside your head. Drop it. Accept it for what it is. Stop asking why.

Possible or maybe?

This is like asking *why*. Your mind will often give you lots of possibilities and lots of different reasons to back up how you are feeling. Stop and get curious about what you are filling your stress bucket with. Is it something that will possibly happen or will maybe happen? Make a promise to yourself to only ever deal with *definitely*. If your Primitive Mind is debating and arguing about whether you need to do something or not, ask yourself whether this is something you possibly need to do? Maybe need to do? Or definitely need to do?

Are you worrying about something possible, maybe or definite? Don't give any attention to things in your mind that are possibles or maybes. When you notice you are giving attention to these... stop. Shake it off and get back on The Now Step®.

Is this easy? Is this simple?

How often in life do you choose the hard option? When you book a holiday abroad does your mind tell you that maybe you should drive four hours to a different airport when your closest airport is thirty minutes away?

When you have a deadline for a presentation and you could update a previous one does your mind tell you to start another one from scratch?

When you are in the supermarket queue with a full trolley and suddenly realise you have forgotten to buy chicken for tonight's dinner, does your mind tell you to come out of the busy queue or to make pasta and meatballs tonight because they are already in your trolley?

What is the easiest and simplest option? What do you normally choose to do? Do you listen to your primitive, negative brain trying to give you more stress? Don't give in.

Always stop and think: Is this easy? Is this simple? If it's not, then do not do it. Always choose the simplest and easiest option.

Other people's behaviour

This can be a difficult one to manage. How often in your day are you met with other people's disappointment, expectations and attitude? You can go out your way to support and be there for some people and it will never be enough. When you find yourself in a situation where someone else's behaviour is affecting you and pulling you off The Now Step®, stop and recognise this.

You will never be able to change how other people are. All you can concentrate on is how you are. To operate from Intellectual Mind control and from your true values, you must be able to let go of situations that upset you. You do you! Walk away from things that don't serve you. You are better than that.

Life will always try and pull you away from The Now Step®. What is happening in your surroundings will always try and pull you away from The Now Step®. Your thoughts in your mind and your body's physiological response to things will always try and pull you away from The Now Step®. Stop... reset... and shake it off.

11

THE CENTRAL NERVOUS SYSTEM

Let's look at the physiology part of the mental wellness framework.

This information changed the game for me in managing my own mental health and I see the penny drop for my clients when they start to learn it. I believe this is information that everyone should know and understand. I think they should teach it in school. I don't mean the central nervous system that is taught in biology, but rather relating it directly to mental health.

It is bad enough when you have all those crazy thoughts and obsessive thinking. Most people suffering mental health issues also experience physical sensations in the body or issues with sleeping at night.

Physical symptoms can show up as:

Palpitations

Tight chest

Racing heart

Shaking

Dizziness

Tingling sensations

Headaches

Migraines

Muscle tension

Aches and soreness

Diarrhoea, constipation

Irritable bowel syndrome

Sleep issues or disorders

If you experience these, this is the normal physiology of how your body works. There is nothing wrong with you, you are not weird, and you are not the only one that feels like this. When one of these symptoms shows up, you certainly don't need to be admitted to hospital. On two or three occasions when my anxiety was off the scale, I took myself to accident and emergency thinking I was having a heart attack and I was going to die. It feels real and very scary. It was stress and anxiety. It can affect your body in many ways.

If you do have any concerns about your health or the way you feel, it is always best to be seen by your GP or a health care professional. You are always better being safe than sorry.

Think about the other bodily sensations you feel in a day. When you have a grumble in your tummy because you have been in nonstop meetings all day and haven't eaten since breakfast, this is normal, right? You don't google, "Why is my stomach making a funny sound?"

What about that itch you had last night and you asked your partner to give it a good scratch? Normal, right? You didn't lie there thinking you must call the GP because your leg was itchy. What about the hiccups? It is such a weird bodily sensation but one that is a very normal physiological response when you get involuntary contractions in your diaphragm. You're certainly not straight away panicking and googling whether hiccups are a sign of cancer.

And think about the last time you did some exercise and got sweaty or went outside and felt cold because you didn't take a jacket. Normal, right? Your body responds to external and internal factors. Your body reacts to its surroundings. It is the normal physiology of how your body works. So there is no need to panic when one of the symptoms in the list above shows up for you.

Health anxiety is a very common mental health condition. I suffered from it myself. Health anxiety is directly linked to how full your stress bucket is. It often shows up in men when they have a full stress bucket. Get your stress bucket under control and as your general anxiety levels come down so too will your health anxiety.

Learning how to manage your mind and not turn those thoughts into thinking is key in managing health anxiety. This runs on a constant cycle of:

- Noticing a bodily sensation or a lump
- Feeling anxious about it
- Experiencing challenging thoughts and catastrophic misinterpretations which you grab onto and turn into thinking (cue crazy lady/man voice)
- Behaviours that temporarily make you feel better like googling, poking and prodding, withdrawing from people, using alcohol to switch off your mind, constant GP visits
- Temporary relief

Then the cycle continues. It is the constant cycle of:

Thoughts = feelings = action = results.

By taking charge of your mind and your thoughts and breaking the cycle, you can help manage your health anxiety. Using The Now Step® method will break the cycle.

Health anxiety is not actually about your body physically but about the relationship you have with your thoughts and your crazy lady/man mind. Similarly, your anxiety is not about the physical symptoms but rather the thoughts you have about the physical symptoms. Crazy right?

Have you ever been in the supermarket and suddenly physically felt weird? Anxious? Perhaps tingly? Maybe you have been asked to present on stage at work and your chest turns red and you feel like you are having a panic attack? Or what about in the hairdressers? Who has felt jittery or just not right when in the hairdressers? Have you ever stopped to wonder why this is?

What do you talk about with your hairdresser? If you are anything like me, you probably tell your hairdresser things that you wouldn't tell anyone else. It is as if there is a secret legion between clients and hairdressers. Think back to your last visit. You can bet your bottom dollar that you were moaning about work, talking about a drama currently happening in your family or how much you hate your partner. All negative chatter. Is it the trip to the hairdressers that makes you have physical symptoms of anxiety? No, it isn't. It is all the negative chatter you have when you get there.

Remember, negative chatter fills your stress bucket. When your stress bucket fills, you go back to anxiety mode. Think about trips to the supermarket or shops. When do you ever go there operating 100% from The Now Step®? Never? You spend the car journey talking through what you are going to buy, how expensive food is, how much you hate food shopping, how much you hate food. And then you arrive at the shop and your mind is whirling at a million miles per hour trying to find the food you want and need. This is all normal. This is your body's physiology responding to what is going on in your mind (the psychology).

I experienced this normal physiology first hand during a recent trip to Alton Towers with my kids. We were at the water park, and I had been on all the water rides. I suddenly started to feel shaky and tingly, the exact same feelings I used to get when I had my anxiety and panic attacks. But I understand all this stuff. I live and breathe The Now Step® mental health management method every day. I knew it was just the adrenaline running through my body with all the excitement. I was able to get on The Now Step®, have Intellectual Mind control and gently remind myself that I was safe, I was calm, I was well, and that this was the normal physiology of how my body works.

Reminding yourself of this the next time you are in a situation when you feel physically unwell. Gently remind yourself that this is the normal physiology of how your body works. You are safe and you are okay. Don't allow your crazy lady/man mind to tell you it's your mental health, because it isn't. Have a quiet word with yourself the next time you feel like this.

Prepare for the meeting or the supermarket trip that you know is going to leave you feeling wound up. Do your *What's been good?* on the journey. Take five minutes in the car before you go rushing in. Give yourself five minutes to breathe.

What is happening is your body's and mind's response to your autonomic nervous system. What follows is information about the two parts of this system. They are the parasympathetic nervous system and the sympathetic nervous system.

This nervous system controls the nerves of the body's inner organs, including your heart, digestion and lungs. You have no conscious control over this.

When the parasympathetic nervous system is activated it produces a calm and relaxed feeling in the mind and body. It controls your bodily functions when you are at rest, it stimulates digestion and your metabolism, and it helps you to relax. Think about it as your 'jammies on and chill' mode. You know that feeling when you get home after a long day and get your comfies on? When you light a candle and have a bath?

Then you have the sympathetic nervous system. When this is activated it stimulates the fight, flight or freeze response inside your amygdala. It is involved in energy expending, enabling the body to use its energy appropriately to respond to dangerous and stressful situations.

Your body floods with stress hormones, boosting your heart rate and sending extra blood to your muscles, lungs and heart. We will call this the 'tiger and run' part of the nervous system. It could also be called 'see an ex-boyfriend and run', 'see an email about a meeting with your boss' or 'kids on summer holidays as you try and work from home' – but for our purpose we will refer to it as 'tiger and run' mode.

The normal physiology of how your body works

We need to investigate in more detail where your physical feelings and sensations of your mental wellness come from. These three modes are very helpful to watch out for in yourself and in colleagues and family members.

Parasympathetic
Sympathetic
Sympathetic shut down

1 Parasympathetic 'jammies on and chill' mode

Signs and symptoms:

Calm and relaxed
Resting and recuperating
Breathing easily
Body feels relaxed

Able to communicate
Processing information easily
Able to tune into environment
Feeling good
Sleeping and eating well

When we operate from our intellectual 'jammies on and chill' part of the brain, life is sweet. We are calm and we love life.

However, let's look at the other two modes.

2 Sympathetic 'tiger and run' mode

Think for a minute about an Indian gazelle munching the grass in the wild. It is minding its own business. And out of the corner of its eye it sees a tiger coming towards it. It has two options. It can fight or take flight. It subconsciously decides whether this is an animal it can fight off. If so, it will go for the kill, but given it's a tiger, the gazelle will decide to run for its life and he will take flight. Both fight and flight are normal physiological responses to help the gazelle stay alive.

Signs and symptoms:

Blood moves around body faster
HR increases
Cortisol and other stress hormones are released
Feeling jittery
Quick reactions/jumpy
Can only process information right here right now
Unable to think rationally
Anxious/angry/puffed up/alert

Can you recognise any of these in yourself? When have you been in fight or flight mode over the past week? Sure, you've not been running away from a tiger, but what has caused you to feel one of these? Running late and stuck in traffic? A fight with your partner? A deadline for a project? Another staff member off sick?

These signs and symptoms are all part of the normal physiology of how your body and mind works. But perhaps you do not accept the emotion or feeling in your body when you feel like this. You then start overthinking, obsessively thinking about why you are feeling jittery, why you are having heart palpitations. You think you are not coping, that your anxiety is out of control, that you need to go and see your GP. Stop. Just stop. This is all normal.

But there is more... what happens when that little gazelle realises that it can't fight the tiger off, nor can it outrun. It only has one option left and that is to freeze. It stays as still as can be in the hope that the tiger gets distracted and loses interest. So here we have fight, flight or freeze mode.

This leads us to a third mode.

3 Sympathetic shut down 'tiger and freeze mode'

Stress overload - need to survive so shuts off systems

Can't move
Dissociation
Dizzy eyes - may feel 'starey'
Feeling sick

Feeling low
Lungs constrict - harder to breathe
Difficulty getting words out/brain fog/procrastination
Body may collapse or want to take up foetal position
Complete overwhelm

When this shows up, you will want to stay in bed. You will not be able to go outside, and you are very likely to phone in sick. This mode is a very scary place to be. It was my default when I was overwhelmed and burned out. Some days I couldn't even remember my phone number or who certain people were. Again, this is the normal physiology of how your body works.

Can you relate to any of the signs or symptoms of the sympathetic shut down mode? Do you recognise any of them in colleagues or family members?

Let's remember the mental wellbeing framework here. There is a constant cycle of your physiology and how you feel which then leads to your psychology and what you are thinking. You feel a sensation in your body and then your mind starts playing games. That crazy lady/man mind starts telling you that you are anxious/depressed or not coping.

What you are feeling is a normal physiological response to the stress of the situation and what is going on in your life. You are not mentally unwell or broken. You can use this knowledge to keep calm and stay in Intellectual Mind control. The more time you spend in Intellectual Mind mode, the less time you spend in primitive survival mode.

Right now, you might not be spending any time in your relaxed 'jammies on and chill' part of your brain but rather running around, afraid to say no to people, constantly stressed and constantly in fight, flight or freeze mode.

The opposite of stressing is relaxing. You can't be stressed and relaxed at the same time.

If there was a scale of 1-10 on the stress scale and 1-10 on the relaxed scale, you can't be a 5 on one and a 3 on the other. It is not possible. You are either stressing or you are relaxing. Agreed?

Since you woke up this morning, how much time have you given to relaxing? Really relaxing. I know it's not possible in the middle of meetings to undress and get your jammies on and go into chill mode, but what have you done that mimics this and makes you feel this way? What have you done today to relax? It could be a ten-minute walk, fifteen minutes to enjoy your lunch without your phone as a distraction, maybe twenty minutes of meditation. How much time have you given to your Intellectual Mind and the 'jammies on and chill' mode? Not much?

Think about how much time you have given today to stressing and being in fight, flight or freeze mode. The minute your alarm goes off your body wakes and stress hormones flood through your body, and then what? Rushing around with the kids? Answering emails as you eat your breakfast? Running from one meeting to the next? If this is your day, you are constantly in stress mode.

When you are in stress mode which part of your brain are you operating from? Your primitive. When you are in your Primitive Mind what are you going to get? Anxiety, depression or anger. You will also get repeated behaviour that takes you into your hippocampus and makes you behave the same way as you did yesterday. This is why you might binge eat or have OCD or have ongoing problems with drinking too much alcohol.

When you are stressed, your mind becomes stressed and busy too. You get even more crazy lady/man thoughts. And the cycle continues.

Can you imagine how you would feel mentally and physically if you gave as much time in a day to relaxing as you do to stressing? Can you imagine how different the *world* would be if we all gave as much time to relaxing as we did stress?

It's up to you what you fill your 24 hours in a day with.

But what can you do when it's not possible to put your jammies on and chill?

Here are my top tips and tools to use throughout the day to increase the time you spend relaxing and reduce the time you spend stressing. Remember, if your mind is still busy and you are constantly off The Now Step® in thinking mode filling your stress bucket then it's not classed as relaxing time.

All these techniques put you into 'jammies on and chill' mode. More importantly, they help stimulate your vagus nerve which is the main nerve of your parasympathetic nervous system. Stimulating it has been shown to reduce anxiety, stress and even depression. When you have a well 'toned' vagus nerve you will be able to relax quicker after stress. The more you practise these exercises and the more toned your vagus nerve becomes, the better your mental health will be. It's almost showing your body an alternative to dealing with stress.

Get practising these:

1 In for four, out for more

Breathing slowly is the simplest way to get back on The Now Step® and switch into the parasympathetic nervous system. My favourite breathing technique is in for four and out for more. Gently close your eyes and drop your shoulders. Unclench your jaw and let your tongue rest lightly at the arch of your mouth. Now gently and slowly breathe in through your nose for the count of four, notice the pause, then breathe out gently through a relaxed mouth for the count of five or six. In for four and out for more. That's it. Nice and easy. You can repeat this as many times as you need depending on how long you have. With each breath allow yourself to relax more and more deeply onto The Now Step®.

2 The grounding technique

This is a great exercise to add into your daily practice as and when you can. You can do it sitting in the car, in the toilets at work or even on a park bench. Have both feet flat on the floor and be in a seated position. Its lovely to do this exercise with bare feet in your back garden or indeed any time you have the opportunity. When you are feeling really stressed find five or ten minutes to do this.

Close your eyes and relax. Begin your breathing in for four and out for more. Now I want you to imagine that you are sitting firmly on The Now Step®. Imagine that coming out of the soles of your feet are big strong roots like those of an old oak tree.

These roots are going to start going down through the earth. They pass through the floor, down through the carpet or grass, down through all the layers of mud and rock, down and down through the lava and all the way to the earth's core, where they wrap themselves around the centre of the earth grounding you and holding you tightly.

You feel safe. You feel grounded. You feel calm. As you continue to imagine the roots tightly fixed around the earth's core and continue to take nice slow gentle breaths, you can gently repeat to yourself: I am calm; I am safe; I am grounded.

You can do this exercise for as long as you want, whether that is two minutes, five minutes or ten minutes. It doesn't matter. The more times you practise this, the more you are switching on your 'jammies on and chill' part of your brain. Prioritise being calm and relaxed.

3 Change your state

When I say change your state, I mean change your physical state, but I also mean change your mental state.

I am sure when you have feelings of anxiety or low mood which show up as physical symptoms, you do feel like you are in a state. It is time to knock yourself out of that state as soon as possible. Continuing to feel like this is doing you no good whatsoever.

I have two things I want you to try. Both will quickly help change your physiological state. You may like one more than the other or they may work differently at different times of the day.

Let's think back again to our little gazelle in India.

When he has escaped the jaws of the tiger, he will automatically give himself a little shake to bring his body back to homeostasis. All animals naturally do this. It's a very normal, natural animal response to shake away fear and stress.

I want you to do the same. For a few minutes I want you to shake your body. Shake your head, your arms, and your legs. Shake, shake, shake off that feeling of energy and adrenaline. You can stand up and shake or you can sit down and shake. Just shake.

I still use this tool every day. I don't fully shake myself anymore, but I do give myself a little internal shudder to remind myself to get back on The Now Step®.

The other thing I want you to try is by moving and talking really slowly. Soooo slowly. Almost like a robot that is in slow mode.

Walk across the room slowly, speak to yourself in the mirror in a slow voice. Go and make a cup of tea but do it so slowly. Do it at snail's pace.

Moving slowly tricks the mind into thinking that the danger has passed. You wouldn't be moving slowly if it was still there. Normally in life you rush around and fly from one thing to the next, which stimulates your stress response. Try being in charge and tricking your mind. Just wait and watch your feelings of stress and anxiety go away.

This is a great trick to use before you sit down to meditate or relax. Allow yourself the transition from your busy day by moving slowly for five minutes before you sit down.

4 The butterfly hug technique

This is a good technique to use if, like me, you are a tactile person. It is a lovely way to self soothe and help you relax. It is a form of bilateral stimulation which calms the nervous system. It can be done anywhere and at any time to move you into 'jammies and chill' mode.

First sit comfortably and imagine yourself on The Now Step®. Take a few slow relaxing breaths. You can close your eyes or keep them open. Cross your arms over your chest so your fingers are gently touching your shoulders. If you want, you can hook your thumbs together. Now begin tapping your hands gently, one at a time. Right, left, right, left, almost like a butterfly tapping its wings. Continue to breathe slowly and keep your jaw and shoulders relaxed.

5 Humming like a bee

Any kind of sound inside your body helps stimulate the vagus nerve.

If you have ever done yoga, you may have done something like this in class. Block your ears with your fingers. This helps to shut out any external noise. Hum. So easy and so effective.

Try all these things out. These tips and tricks will allow you to switch into 'jammies and chill mode' even as you go about your busy day. Find out which ones help you the most and make you feel the calmest. The more you practise, the easier they will become, and they will soon be part of your normal daily routine.

12

THE NOW STEP® EYES OPEN MEDITATION

Meditation is probably the one thing that I can say well and truly changed my life, my understanding about my mind and my mental health.

When I was in the depths of despair with my mental health, I associated myself with anxiety. I was anxiety. I was all my crazy nonstop thoughts. It was a dark and frightening time for me. When you see yourself as that crazy voice in your head who always thinks the worst, it sucks all the joy and happiness out of your day.

Even if you think meditation is too woowoo and fluffy cloud, please bear with me. I have developed The Now Step® eyes open and eyes closed meditation just for you. It is practical and matter of fact and you can do it as you go about your busy life.

Meditation allows you to have five or ten minutes in a day when you are still. It is an excuse in a busy world to be able to sit down and switch off. It is a selfless way to have ten or twenty minutes of stillness and relaxation. It brings so many benefits to your mental and physical health. It reduces stress and can improve symptoms of stress-related illnesses like IBS and headaches.

It can:

Improve memory and give you better focus
Increase attention
Improve willpower – helping strengthen the mental discipline to stay away from unwanted habits and compulsive behaviours.
Improve sleep
Reduce pain and inflammation
Lower blood pressure – during meditation your blood pressure drops and over time this can reduce strain on the heart and prevent heart disease
Reduce anxiety
Lessen depression
Enhance compassion
Give you time alone with your thoughts

At first the idea of having time alone in your head can seem daunting and rather scary, especially when your mind is full of anxious, worst-case scenario and repetitive thoughts. If you suffer from OCD and constant thoughts on overdrive, the idea of sitting with your mind can seem counter intuitive. When you first give it a go and try to switch off, it can feel like the hardest thing in the world. Have you ever tried it? Perhaps you already meditate daily? Or perhaps you have given it a go only to have sat there and felt even more stressed when you became aware of just how crazy and busy your mind is.

But that is the beauty and simplicity in this. You are not trying to get rid of your thoughts. You are just trying to begin to notice them. You are trying to become aware of them coming and going.

It is a bit like a train coming into the station and you choosing whether to get on or not. You have a choice.

The Now Step® eyes open meditation is one of the simplest ways to add meditation into your busy life. Yes, you got that right, eyes *open* meditation. There is no need to sit cross-legged in lotus position or in a dark, quiet room. There is no need to take time out of your busy schedule to meditate. With The Now Step® eyes open meditation you can get all the benefits of meditation as you go about your day.

Just like using *What's been good?* to stop turning those thoughts into thinking, you can use this tool to help you stay on The Now Step® and keep your stress bucket empty.

As you go about your day, when you are driving your car, when you are between work meetings, as you lie in the bath or have a shower, you can use The Now Step® eyes open meditation to help keep your stress bucket empty. The next time you book a massage or lie on your sunbed on holiday, you can use The Now Step® eyes open meditation to stop turning those thoughts into thinking.

The first thing you need to do is find one or two anchoring statements that are called your Now Step mottos. These are going to be your own powerful messages to your subconscious mind. Choose whatever resonates with you.

They will help you get all the above mental and physical benefits from meditating. It will be your own way to stop you thinking and going over the same things time and time again. It will remind you to stop... reset... and get back on The Now Step®. It will help you to break away from the chatter with your crazy lady or crazy man.

Your Now Step motto must be something easy to remember that makes you feel uplifted and empowered. It must be something that gives direct positive suggestion to your subconscious mind.

Let me give you some suggestions:

I can and I will. (This is my go to.)
I love me.
I am safe.
I am calm.
I am successful.
I have my dream job.
I choose peace.
I choose love.
I choose The Now Step®.
I deserve happiness and love.
I deserve the best.
I deserve rest.
Thank you for my good health.
I am enough.
The past is useless.

If even these seem too airy-fairy and fluffy cloud, choose something more factual.

I love motorbikes.
I love Liverpool FC.
I love baking.
I am strong.
I am Lyn.
I am respected.
I choose a latte.
I choose to go to the gym.
I choose me.

It doesn't matter what you say. What matters is that it is uplifting, and that when you say it, it slips easily off your tongue and will ground you back onto The Now Step® like an anchor. All the motto is doing is reminding you to stop turning those thoughts into thinking.

I want you to set your timer on your phone for five minutes and practise this with your eyes closed to begin with. You can do this lying down, in the bath or sitting up on your bed. There are no rules.

It is similar to the way that you did the counting your thoughts exercise. This time, rather than give your thoughts a number every time you notice one, I want you to gently say the motto you have chosen every time you notice yourself thinking.

Close your eyes and imagine yourself firmly stuck on The Now Step®, using Intellectual Mind control. Relax your shoulders and breathe out. Relax. Begin to watch your mind.

When you notice a thought, gently say to yourself the motto you have chosen such as, "I can, and I will."

Notice yourself on The Now Step® in Intellectual Mind control. Notice the pause or the space that is in your mind right now. Watch your mind move and a thought come up.

Again, at this point that you notice the thought, gently say your motto. Perhaps you will begin to drift away and turn one of the thoughts into thinking. That is okay. That is normal. All that matters is that there is a point that you notice you are doing this and stop yourself. It might be you notice a thought or that you have turned the thought into thinking. Again, at this point gently say your motto.

Allow your shoulders to relax again and keep breathing gently. Sit on The Now Step® in Intellectual Mind control. And repeat.

Say The Now Step® motto you have chosen as many times as you need to in the five minutes. You don't want to be chanting out the motto again and again. Just say it gently when you notice you are thinking.

When you first begin to practise, you may find some resistance to doing it. This is all normal. Your crazy lady/crazy man voice will show up to remind you of all the other jobs you have to do in the house and telling you that this exercise is pointless. They will try to distract you in every way possible. They want you to self-sabotage and stop doing it. They want to pull you off The Now Step® and back into the survival negative part of your brain.

But you get to choose! This is five minutes when your Intellectual Mind is in control, when you are aware of those thoughts coming in but choosing not to engage with them. You choose to watch for the pause and the space between all the ongoing thoughts. This space is The Now Step®.

This is gold dust brain training and the quickest way to strengthen your Intellectual Mind, giving you better mental wellness.

Massive congratulations on doing your first five minutes of meditation, spending five minutes giving your attention to the part of you that matters. Well done for prioritising you.

To begin with, aim to give five minutes twice a day to this activity. Perhaps sit up in bed once your alarm has gone off, use your lunch break or use it to help relax you at bedtime. After a few weeks, try doing it for ten minutes two or three times a day.

Remember, you can do this anywhere that you can close your eyes. On a park bench, travelling on a train or while getting a massage.

You can also add in a second motto. You can either say motto one for five minutes then switch to motto two for five minutes or you can set a timer for ten minutes and alternate your motto every time you notice a thought or notice that you are away in thinking mode.

There is no right or wrong way to do this. Take just ten minutes to allow yourself to be on The Now Step®, in Intellectual Mind control, not filling your stress bucket.

Ten minutes in 'jammies and chill' mode where your parasympathetic nervous system is getting a chance to relax and recuperate.

Make your mental health your priority and give ten minutes two or three times a day to this. Your brain and body will thank you for it and you will see huge benefits as the days go on. No excuses. Just do it.

Now you have the hang of doing this with your eyes closed it is super easy to start doing it as you go about your day when your eyes are open. You can use it as another way to stay on The Now Step® and not fill up your stress bucket.

Every time you catch yourself off The Now Step® and turning those thoughts into thinking, chatting away with your crazy lady or man voice, gently say your motto internally. Say whichever one slips off your tongue easily. Then repeat; it is that easy. When you are out for a walk today and you notice you are off The Now Step®... gently say your motto. When you are driving to work and you're not actually there in the car but chatting negatively to crazy lady or man... gently say your motto. When you bump into your negative neighbour and you feel your mind being drawn into negative conversation... gently say your motto.

When you are in a meeting at work and the negativity and drama starts and you feel your Primitive Mind racing... gently say your motto. When you are sitting on a bench looking over at a wonderful view and your mind starts thinking... gently say your motto. When you are in the shower in the morning... use your eyes open meditation.

Anywhere, any time of the day when your eyes are open you can immediately bring yourself back onto The Now Step® by internally saying your motto.

"I can and I will."

"I love me."

"I am safe."

Whatever works for you. Whatever stops your thinking in its tracks. Whatever brings you back onto The Now Step®.

By using both the eyes open as you go about your day and your eyes closed The Now Step® meditation, you will begin to see the joy and simplicity of present moment living.

It is where you don't talk negatively or get involved in drama. It is where you don't go over things that happened three days ago. It is where you don't waste any moments of your precious life fretting about the future.

It is where you are in control of your mind.

You are perfect and whole exactly as you are.

13

HORMONES AND MENTAL HEALTH

If you are a male reading this, please don't skip past this chapter. There is information in here about both sexes and how hormones affect your mental health.

I am also sure you have many women in your life, whether a daughter, wife, friend or colleague and you would benefit from having more understanding of their hormones too.

Hormones in woman play a vital role in their reproductive system. They also play havoc with their mood, motivation, energy levels and mental health.

If you are still in the reproductive years, you will recognise times in the month that you feel on top of the world. You will have days that you feel your mental health and your anxiety is much worse. You may feel good for a few days and then suddenly your anxiety is back. It can often leave you feeling deflated and questioning if you will ever be able to live anxiety free. You must believe me – yes, you can!

The reason your anxiety or depression can feel worse at different times of the month is due to the female sex hormone progesterone. Progesterone is released by the corpus luteum in the ovaries and plays an important role in the menstrual cycle and the early stages of pregnancy. Levels of progesterone peak twice in your monthly cycle. They peak around the time you ovulate (roughly day fourteen of your cycle) and then peak again 24-48 hours before menstruation begins.

Progesterone stimulates the amygdala. We spoke about the amygdala in Chapter Three when we spoke about your brain. The amygdala is situated in the Primitive Brain and is where your fight, flight or freeze response comes from.

Progesterone stimulates the amygdala and your anxiety. This is the reason that halfway through your cycle and on the days leading up to your period you may notice your anxiety is worse. It is the physiology of how your body works so be prepared for this. Don't allow your crazy lady to go crazy during these days. Calmly remind yourself that there is a physiological reason that you feel so bad. Make sure you are working extra hard to stay on The Now Step®. Make your self-care and time to be in 'jammies and chill' mode a priority.

During the peri-post menopausal years (age 38-54) you no longer have an equilibrium of hormones in your body.

Therefore, some days you can feel better than others. The constant changes in your hormones can result in you feeling anxious, constantly overthinking, feelings of depression, low self-worth, and lost confidence. Physical symptoms can show up as heart palpitations, changes in body temperature and gut health and your sleep can be affected. During this time, you can't deal with stress as effectively as you did ten years ago. It becomes a constant battle and vicious cycle.

When you have ongoing stress, your body maintains high levels of cortisol throughout the day. Over a period of months, this can have a detrimental effect on you both physically and emotionally. It can lead to adrenal fatigue.

The adrenal glands are small triangular glands located on top of both kidneys. Their job is to produce hormones that regulate metabolism, the immune system, blood pressure and more importantly your response to stress.

During menopause the ovaries stop working and stop producing progesterone and oestrogen, and the adrenal glands then take over the production of these hormones.

However, when you are always stressed the adrenal glands are required to produce constant cortisol and this takes over from them producing the two hormones progesterone and oestrogen. So, managing your stress levels during this time is so important to allow the adrenal glands to effectively produce the correct balance of hormones.

Stress is such a subjective thing and often comes into your life without you asking for it, perhaps because of ill health, a relationship breakdown or financial worries. Most of the stress, however, is brought on by the relationship you have with your mind... how you think about these situations and how much you are off The Now Step®.

During perimenopause stress management is very important and this begins with you managing your mind.

Things that can also help:

1. Sleep (using a nightly hypnosis can help massively)
2. Relaxation (breathing, meditating, yoga)
3. Balancing blood sugars (cut sugar and alcohol from your diet)
4. No caffeine (decaf tea and coffee always)
5. Supplements (e.g. magnesium, vitamin C and D, vitamin B12)
6. Moving your body (walking and some gentle body weight exercises are ideal)

Use these questions to check in with yourself:

1. How many hours of constant sleep did you get last night?
2. How much time today have you spent relaxing?
3. How much sugar did you consume today?
4. How much caffeine have you had today?
5. What supplements did you take today?
6. What movement have you done today?
7. Have you been on The Now Step® today?

Sleep and early morning anxiety

It's Monday morning and you have the busiest day ahead of you with meetings every hour on the hour.

The minute your alarm goes off that feeling of doom and panic and the horrible knot in your stomach is there. You haven't even been in the shower yet and already you are feeling anxious and you fear getting through the day.

You feel tired all the time but can't get a decent night's sleep and your confidence is at an all-time low. Welcome to the perimenopause.

And that feeling of anxiety first thing in the morning? It's not the way you want to start your day.

There are two main things that cause morning anxiety.

The first thing is cortisol.

When your body is under stress it produces cortisol and adrenaline. These are the fight, flight or freeze hormones and are needed to keep you alive and safe. In our cave days they were there to help you flee from the tiger. They gave you energy, focus and made you alert. In modern days the scary tiger now equates to a new job, a breakdown in a relationship and all the daily politics going on in the office.

Cortisol's main job is to:

1. Increase your blood sugar and your energy
2. Stabilise your blood pressure
3. Reduce inflammation

It is needed to get you up in the morning, ready and alert to face the day full of energy and motivated to deal with 'the tiger'.

Cortisol is produced in a cycle and is highest in the morning and should reduce as the day goes on, so that you are ready at bedtime for sleep. This cycle is called the Cortisol Awakening Response (CAR).

It is a normal physiological cycle in your body. For the first 30-45 minutes when you first wake up, it is normal to feel this energy and alertness. (Can you imagine the size of the knot in your stomach when 'the tiger' is pouncing at you.) But this early morning physical feeling interferes with your ability to think calmly and to plan for the day ahead. It makes you think, "I am anxious."

As we go into our peri-post menopausal years our hormones are all over the place and this changes the way we respond to stress. Therefore, the morning anxiety feels worse now than ten years ago. It's the effect of cortisol. It is normal. That's why managing your stress is so important.

The second thing is your crazy lady mind.

The minute your alarm goes off in the morning, there she is catastrophising and ruining your day. It becomes a negative cycle. You wake up and cortisol is higher so you 'feel' anxious. Then crazy lady starts you 'thinking' you are anxious. And on and on it goes.

Tomorrow morning when you wake up, give this a go:

1. Gently remind yourself that this feeling in the morning is normal. That it is cortisol.
2. Don't lie in bed chatting to your crazy lady voice. Get up.

3. For one or two minutes shake your body. Shake off the adrenaline and cortisol, like you are running away from 'the tiger'.
4. Then move really, really slowly. Like the slowest you can move. Don't rush to get the kids up or rush to get in the shower. S-L-O-W-L-Y. Go to the bathroom or to the kitchen to make a coffee (and please make sure it's a decaf coffee. Caffeine is the worst thing for morning anxiety.)
5. For the first twenty minutes in the morning go *slow*. Fill the kettle. Have your shower. Perhaps sit down for that time and breathe or meditate. Nothing else.
6. Keep reminding yourself gently that you are safe, you are well and that what you are feeling is the normal physiology of how your body works.
7. Do not pour your crazy lady a coffee or let her into the shower with you. This is *your* time.

How hormones affect men

It's not only woman who are affected by hormones.

Look at the raging hormones in teenage boys. Hormone surges during puberty can cause mood swings, anger and irritability in boys. Suddenly your sweet twelve-year-old turns into a raging bull who slams doors and gets angry at the smallest thing. The changing level in the hormone testosterone is responsible for this.

Low levels of testosterone can cause depression, anxiety, or other mental health conditions in men.

There is something medically known and recognised as 'the male menopause'. Men in their late 40s and early 50s can develop depression and other emotional symptoms. They can have mood swings, a lack of energy or enthusiasm, tiredness and difficulty sleeping, and short-term memory loss. It is believed that it is not actually dropping levels of testosterone that causes this. Although testosterone levels decrease as a man gets older, it is often lifestyle choices and stress that causes their mental health to decline. Men must prioritise both their physical and mental wellbeing. Stress management plays a huge role in this.

Changing hormones can affect both men's and women's mental health. However, it is often the lack of understanding about managing your mind that causes you to feel anxious, stressed and depressed.

Using The Now Step® mental health management method can help you to manage your mind and stay in control despite all the changes in hormones.

14

HOW TO BE SOLUTION-FOCUSED

Using solution-focused questions and learning how to ask yourself solution-focused questions is a powerful way to help you stay mentally well.

When you have a day of low mood or perhaps feeling unmotivated, they really help you to refocus and look at small steps you can take. When your mental health is not great and you are generally not feeling on top of everything, the thought of long to do lists and big goals can be well and truly overwhelming. When I discovered how much solution-focused questioning and looking at things in a solution-focused way helped me, it was life changing. No more fixating on the problem. "What can I do to stop myself feeling anxious?" turned into, "What one small step can I take today to feel calm and relaxed?"

Using solution-focused questions with my clients is always lots of fun, whether that is in group sessions or one-to-one. And why is it fun? Because they are not thinking about negative things.

I can see the 'cogs turning' in their brains and the exact moment when they realise that thinking in this way stops the primitive crazy lady or man mind in its tracks and switches on intellectual positive mind control.

When you begin to use solution-focused questions, and especially when you start using The Now Step® mental health management method, you may find it challenging to answer these types of questions. This is because the negative part of your brain is in charge. The crazy lady doesn't want you imagining your preferred future. It wants to keep you stuck in survival mode. But you are better than that. You are way stronger than that. You can become positive and solution-focused.

The more times you use solution-focused questions, the stronger your mind muscles become and the easier you find it. You begin to become more solution-focused and more positive about everything in your life. Clients leave sessions with me feeling happy and motivated because they have been the expert in that time, and they have taken control of which good things they can do more of. How would you rather spend an hour? Talking to me about the drama and awful experiences you have had in the past or about your achievements and your strengths that have made you what you are today? An hour drudging through past painful memories or an hour imagining your perfect, happy and fulfilled future? It is a fun way to navigate life and your mental health.

Already in this book you have learned some solution-focused questions such as *What's been good?* and *What can I do today to get my positive action/interaction?* You can use these questions every day. They are the gold dust solution-focused questions that you need.

These questions give you Intellectual Mind control which encourages you to be in the positive and happy and mentally well part of your brain. This stops you filling your stress bucket and keeps you on The Now Step®.

There are so many solution-focused questions I use during sessions with clients that I could write another book. In this book I have given you the questions that are easiest to use yourself to manage your mind.

Being solution-focused isn't about the questions. It's about the decision you make about how you want your life and your outlook to be. You must be able to flip the switch inside your brain, just like you would change the station on the radio from sad tunes to happy tunes. You can do the same with your mind. The questions only help to support this. Stop focusing on the problem. Become obsessed with the solution. It is your solution to being happy and mentally well.

Problem-focused versus solution-focused questions

Let's look at some examples of problem-focused questions and solution-focused questions. Which do you use more than the other?

Problem focused	Solution focussed
How are you feeling today?	What's been good today?
What does your depression stop you doing?	What can you do to feel happy this week?
What is upsetting you?	What would you like your life to be like?
Why do you hate your job so much?	What would make you enjoy your job?
What has been triggering your OCD?	What have you been doing to stop turning those thoughts into thinking?

The key is to move away from negative words. Stop moaning and talking negatively. Don't sit and chat for hours with your mates about the problem. Be the one who moves the conversation towards positive and solution-focused things. Make sure your internal and external dialogues are not negative.

The important thing to remember here is that it is okay to daydream and imagine your future and come off The Now Step® if you are using positive thinking. It is fine to imagine your preferred future. Your stress bucket only fills with negative thinking.

Daydreaming in a positive way can help you to relax and your mind to take a break from reality and all the worry. Visualisation, done in a positive way, helps you change the brain's function and make more positive neural connections to the Intellectual Mind. It is good for calming anxiety. It helps to take you away from all the negativity and stories inside your head.

This is one of my favourite stories to use with clients as a guided meditation. It allows them to see their preferred future rather than all the crazy, negative nonsense.

Before you read this story take a nice slow breath in and relax your jaw and shoulders. Give your mind permission to follow this story but also to daydream and take from it the powerful subconscious message.

Let's begin...

Once there was a village in a very isolated part of the world. So isolated that the people of the village rarely saw visitors from the outside world. These people had a secret.

They had a magical painting which had been given to them by a stranger in a time before anyone could remember. The stranger had said, "As long as this picture stays in the village, everything will go right for the people of the village." The people felt safe because they had this picture.

One day another stranger came to the village. The hospitable villagers made the stranger welcome and let him stay in the room where the painting was kept, but when they woke in the morning, the stranger had left and the painting was gone.

The villagers were devastated. Their happiness had gone and life could never again be the way they had pictured it. The blue sky had turned dark, the trees had stopped blooming, the birds no longer sang, and they felt very sad.

Then one young woman walked over to the space where the painting had been, and she started to paint her own picture on the wall. She started to paint beautiful trees and birds. Others joined her and soon all the people were co-operating in making this painting. They all became so absorbed in their painting that it wasn't until the young woman looked out of the window and said, "Look! Everything is changing," that they realised the sky had become blue again, and the birds were singing again, and the trees were back in bloom. (anon)

Using a story and language like this helps you to daydream and visualise in a positive, solution-focused way.

What do you want your new painting to look like? How do you imagine your preferred future?

Give yourself five minutes to visualise this.

Solution-focused questions are designed to get answers that are solution-focused. It's one of my favourite things about the work that I do. Being able to use questions to change your brain, your mental health, and the way you see yourself is powerful.

During sessions with clients my job is to help you learn how to be more solution-focused and for you to live from The Now Step®. I show you how to empty your stress bucket with solution-focused techniques. You can then take what you learn and use it after our sessions.

You can start to implement all this stuff yourself. You choose to be solution-focused. You become solution-focused. The changes in every area of your life when you become solution focused are phenomenal. To every problem there is always a solution.

These are three of my favourite solution-focused techniques. Practise using them every day.

1 Scaling

Use a scale from 1-10 where one is being ready to jump off a bridge/your worst version of yourself and ten is being the best version of yourself and giving big woohoos.

You can use scaling regarding anything:

On a scale of 1-10 how confident am I feeling today?

On a scale of 1-10 how happy am I about my career?

On a scale of 1-10 how am I feeling right now?

Using a scale takes away all the emotion and opportunity for the negative crazy lady/man voice and helps you to be intellectually minded.

If you are feeling a five right now, what could you do to be a six? If you are a three on the confidence scale right now, what would make you a four? Always just go one point above. Take small steps towards your goal of being a ten.

Think about a time in your life when you have scored the highest. Allow yourself to daydream and visualise what was going on in your life at that moment. Who were you with? What were you doing? What were you wearing? What was making you feel so good?

Use some of these answers to help move you back up the scale towards being your best version.

2- The miracle question

Let's imagine that when you finish reading this book today that a miracle has happened. I have given my little magic fairy wand a wave and you have your miracle. The minute you go back into your daily life you don't know that there has been a miracle; all you know is that you feel different. You feel better.

Life feels better. The miracle has moved you one point higher up on your scale. You are now a seven rather than a six.

Stop... get on The Now Step®... use Intellectual Mind control. You are a definite seven.

What do you notice that is different about your life, mood or surroundings? How do you feel? How are you holding your body? If your partner walked in the room, what would they notice about you? What would your children notice?

Choose some words that describe what you notice about being a seven rather than a six.

More relaxed, calmer, smiling more, happier, motivated? What word or words came up for you?

Then choose your word. Perhaps you would choose *motivated*. What small step can you take right now that is going to move you towards the wonderful goal of feeling more motivated?

Perhaps you would wash the dishes, go for a run, get the kids away to bed... whatever works for you and is going to make you feel more motivated.

Decide what would make you feel more motivation and then just do it! Do not engage with the negative crazy lady/man mind telling you not to bother. Just do it.

Take one tiny step towards your goal of being a seven rather than a six. Take one little step towards being the best version of yourself.

3- New Year's party

Let's imagine it is New Year's Eve and because you and I are now good friends you invite me along to your New Year's party. We are having the best time, all your close family and friends are there, we are in a lovely venue, whether that is your back garden, a five-star hotel or up a mountain in a ski resort. You choose. The fireworks have just finished and we pour another glass of lovely champagne. We are well and truly having a now step moment.

I put my hand on your shoulder and smile at you. I ask you this question, "What successes have you had this year that have brought you to this moment?"

What do you reply with? What do you tell me? What have your biggest wins and successes been? What have you done this year that has made your heart sing? What have you achieved this year that you are celebrating right now? It might be career wise. It might be financial. Have you met the man of your dreams?

Do it right now. Allow your mind to daydream, imagine and visualise.

This is your reality. These are the possibilities that you must make. You can make them as big or as small as you want.

This preferred future that you are imagining right now at the end of this year can become your reality. You don't have to wait until you are older, fitter or richer. You can choose this reality right now.

What story do you want to be telling when this year ends?

Will the year be full of problems or full of solutions?

After all there is a solution to every problem.

Solution-focused questions allow you to be in control and imagine your preferred future. You get to choose not your therapist.

CONCLUSION

This is one of my favourite quotes of all time. I had it printed on the menus at my fortieth birthday celebration:

> "Life should not be a journey to the grave with the intention of arriving safely in a pretty and well-preserved body, but rather to skid in sideways, thoroughly used up, totally worn out and proclaiming woohoo what a ride."
>
> — ADAPTED FROM HUNTER S THOMPSON

What are you doing to make sure your life is one huge, woohoo, fabulous ride?

If this isn't your wakeup call, then what will be? Life isn't happening tomorrow or next week. It sure is not living in the past. Right here, right now is the only moment you have that matters. Here in the now.

You need to choose to feel mentally well. No one else can do it for you. The solution is not out there somewhere. You are the solution.

One of my incredible members of The Female Mind Retreat is currently battling a brain tumour. I want to share with you her story that she has kindly shared in her own words. Nata is the most inspirational woman I have ever met. I am very honoured to have met her.

We can all get dragged down at times and find life a struggle. We all have our times when life is tougher than others. I hope Nata's story will inspire you as much as it inspires me.

"When I joined Lyn Penman's membership, I already felt at the point of no return… knee deep in plans, self-help books and a mind that wanted to beat the world record for fastest route to nowhere. I knew something had to change or nowhere would be my destination. I was in search of the simple lightbulb moment and here it was in the shape of this bright, down to earth person on my screen. Lyn's brain training techniques and The Now Step® method excited me. From the beginning it felt so interesting, smart, and super easy to put into practice. Maybe I could teach this wild and wandering head of mine that slow and steady wins the race!

Life felt so much better. I was armed with my newfound sense of direction, I had confidence in everything and my priorities were set. I felt I was in control and enjoying life again.

But it was all about to change.

I answered the phone one day. My results were back from the hospital. I was thrown a curveball in the shape of a brain tumour on my left frontal lobe.

It turned out that the knowledge I had gained from Lyn up to this moment was preparing me for the biggest challenge of my life. I felt huge gratitude that somehow Lyn and I had crossed paths at that exact time.

This news could have floored me. I could have been defeated by what I was about to face and how long I would be lucky enough to face it all for. The fear and the worry. But anxiety and worries didn't have the chance to beat me at the race. I was prepared for them.

I remember as a kid the days feeling long and delicious. We delighted in our push pops and were so caught up in the moment that nothing else mattered. Yet as an adult, how did 9pm come round so fast? I lost the ability to keep my feet planted firmly where they needed to be. Instead, they were taking me everywhere but. The days would speed by and there was no way to stop it from happening. Life was flying past me.

Equipped with my newfound mindset and the positivity that came with it, I faced brain surgery and all the mammoth choices I needed to make with a strength I would never have imagined before. I continued to turn my life around.

Now, thanks to Lyn, I delight in the simple things. In a conversation, a smile, a cool drink, and a comfy bed.

Despite my diagnosis and uncertainty about my future, I'm so happy. I can save my mind from anything not in its best interests and have convinced it to stop sprinting. And I have Lyn to thank for this.

My mind is right here where it needs to be.

I am so ready for any challenges heading my way. Life likes to keep us on our toes, but the sweetest part is the process. I feel like I've magically slowed down time... by learning what Lyn has taught me.

The Now Step® is what you need to change your life"

— NATA

How inspirational is Nata? Faced with such a difficult time in life she is still able to find joy. She is the perfect example of present moment living. She is the perfect example of being solution-focused.

You too have this choice. You too can choose to live your life like this. Regardless of what is going on around you. Regardless of what life throws at you.

It is all in your mindset.

You can choose for Intellectual Mind control. You can choose to train your brain to be happy. You can choose to not turn your thoughts into thinking. You can choose to do your daily *What's been good?*

You can choose to do your three Ps every day. You can choose to spend more time in 'jammies and chill' mode. You can choose to disengage from that crazy voice in your head.

You can choose to walk away from relationships and people that bring you down. You can choose not to get involved in drama and negative conversations. You can choose to keep your stress bucket empty. You can choose to be solution-focused.

You can choose to never go over the past. You can choose not to go into the future.

You choose.

On the day of my Dad's funeral in 2006 Mr Mundie the Minister gave me some advice. He walked over to me and put his hands on my shoulders. And he said to me "Lyn, whatever you do in life just make sure you always look up."

It didn't matter to me what my religious beliefs were about heaven. His words allowed me to stop….take a breath…..and look up….taking myself away from the emotions and upset of the moment.

It was a reminder to me that despite all the difficult challenges we face here on earth there is a much bigger picture. That we are tiny in comparison to the vast universe.

You don't need to look into the future because it never comes. You don't need to look into the past because its gone. All you need to do is keep your feet firmly on The Now Step® and remind yourself to always look up.

Never fight your future and never fight your past. But rather show up for life on The Now Step®, and accept it exactly as it is.

Using the techniques learned in this book you can have the life you desire. Calm, contented, happy and mentally well.

You can and you will. You can and you will. Yes, you can and you will.

WITH GRATITUDE

I want to say a special thank you to my clients past, present, and future. It has been an honour to share with you this life-changing way to manage mental health.

I will forever be grateful to the Clifton Practice and in particular Alex Brounger and Anne Wyatt for teaching me the basics of solution-focused work and the skill to be able to help clients work out their own preferred future.

To Sandy Newbigging for being my first spiritual guru and such a beacon of light for me and others.

To my members of The Female Mind Retreat, thank you for taking the step to change your life. I am truly blessed to have you all in my life and now have some of the best friends a girl could ask for. A special thank you to Lindsey.

To my Mum and Jim and my big sister Nichola, who have supported me and been there no matter what, I love you unconditionally.

To my dad, whom we lost in 2006, there is not a day that goes by that I don't think of you. Love you for eternity.

To my best friends forever, Kerry, Sam, and Vicky. Your friendship is everything to me and I am so grateful you are by my side.

To Susan. Thank you for being there to make me smile and laugh so hard that it hurts. It takes someone else with four kids to understand just how hard it is.

To all my school mum pals, my childhood friends and the new friends I have made along the way, thank you for being part of my journey.

To Si, thank you for being the wind beneath my wings. You are a true gentleman. I love you.

To my precious children, Jimmy, Katie, Robby and Toby, thank you for showing me what true love means. This book is for you. May you read and use it as you grow up. May you share with your children and grandchildren. Hear my voice as you read it. I am forever with you. No matter how far apart we are, I am always in your heart. I will always feel blessed that your Dad and I brought you into this world.

You are my reason for waking up in the morning. My reason for living. My reason for writing this book. My world. My everything. I love you all to the moon and back.

WORK WITH ME

Thank you for choosing to read my book. You won't find a better way to understand your mind and manage your mental health. It is the solution that you have been searching for.

If you would like more support in managing your mental health, please reach out to me. I would love to hear how you are getting on implementing The Now Step® method into your life. If you need extra support and are intrigued to explore solution-focused therapy further, then please get in touch.

If you are looking to implement a new mental wellbeing strategy into your corporate organisation then please contact me to discuss. I am also available for keynote and conference events.

My email is lyn@lynpenman.com or I can be contacted via Facebook or LinkedIn.

CPSIA information can be obtained
at www.ICGtesting.com
Printed in the USA
LVHW081109180922
728595LV00012B/225/J